The Moral Distress Syndrome Affecting Physicians

The Moral Distress Syndrome Affecting Physicians

How Current Healthcare Is Putting Doctors and Patients at Risk

Eldo E. Frezza, MD, MBA, FACS

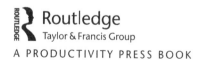

Routledge
Taylor & Francis Group

A PRODUCTIVITY PRESS BOOK

First published 2021
by Routledge
52 Vanderbilt Avenue, New York, NY 10017

and by Routledge
2 Park Square, Milton Park, Abingdon, Oxon, OX14 4RN
Routledge is an imprint of the Taylor & Francis Group, an informa business

---

Library of Congress Cataloging-in-Publication Data

Names: Frezza, Eldo E., author.
Title: The moral distress syndrome affecting physicians : how current healthcare is putting doctors and patients at risk / Eldo E. Frezza.
Description: New York, NY : Routledge, 2021. | Includes bibliographical references and index.
Identifiers: LCCN 2020012901 (print) | LCCN 2020012902 (ebook) | ISBN 9780367473044 (hardback) | ISBN 9780367471538 (paperback) | ISBN 9781003034766 (ebook)
Subjects: MESH: Physicians--psychology | Burnout, Professional--psychology | Psychological Distress
Classification: LCC R690 (print) | LCC R690 (ebook) | NLM WA 495 | DDC 158.7/23--dc23
LC record available at https://lccn.loc.gov/2020012901
LC ebook record available at https://lccn.loc.gov/2020012902

ISBN: 978-0-367-47304-4 (hbk)
ISBN: 978-0-367-47153-8 (pbk)
ISBN: 978-1-003-03476-6 (ebk)

Typeset in Garamond
by Deanta Global Publishing Services, Chennai, India

To all the physicians who are suffering
in silence and in the dark.

To all involved in healthcare systems who are
forgetting that physicians are their customers.
Satisfied physicians produce satisfied patients.

To my children Edoardo and Gianmarco, who
have witnessed a lot in their young age.

Contents

About the Author

Eldo E. Frezza was born and raised in Venice, went to medical school in Italy, and completed his postgraduate course as a resident in the USA. He also obtained a Master's in Business Administration from Texas Tech University. He is a Fellow of the American College of Surgeons (FACS), American Medical Association, and American Medical Physician Leadership. He is now Chief of Surgery at Nashville General Hospital.

An award-winning physician executive who elevates organizational performance and aligns physicians with the rapidly changing healthcare landscape, Eldo E. Frezza is the CEO and founder of Cure Your Practice (www.cureyourpractice.com), has over 40 years of experience providing consulting services to healthcare organizations in the areas of metrics, supply chains, clinical service line development, organizational strategy, alignment, and network formation. This includes healthcare systems, academic medical centers, physician groups, insurance companies, and government agencies, as well as professional organizations.

As medical director of quality and vice president of medical affairs, he has guided the boardroom decision-making that has defined the priorities and direction of many leading healthcare organizations to maintain high quality and ethical values.

The author of three essential textbooks on ethics, business, and laparoscopic surgery, and numerous articles on clinical practice, research, economics, and ethics, Eldo is also authoring books on sociology and fiction. He has published eight books and more than 200 articles in peer-reviewed journals and book chapters. His bestselling book is a diet book, which continues to sell ten years after the second edition was published.

Eldo has been writing books for his classes and continues to be tested by his students. He has always been working on motivation and how to make society better by teaching, showing, and explaining the basic principles of societal ethics, civic responsibility, and wellness. With increasing burnout and suicide among medical students, residents, and doctors, he developed national talks and research on moral distress for the Texas Medical Association, and now he is placing his experience in this book.

He has been a full professor and professor of ethics in several institutions, including Texas A&M, Texas Tech, University of Pittsburgh, etc., and he won several writing contests. He is a regular speaker on ethics, sociology, and medicine for different medical societies and editor of medical journals. Dr. Frezza started as a journalist before going to medical school. He speaks three languages and is often considered a Renaissance man since his background spans medical specialties into ethics, business, sociology, and philosophy. He also served as commander of the Texas Medical Rangers for West Texas.

Why Write This Book?

The information contained in this book is correct to the best of the author's knowledge at the date of publication. The characters, names, and situations are fictional and are in no way meant to report on real people. It is a fiction built around life situations without pointing the finger at anyone specific. The author and publisher assume no liability for damage arising from errors or omissions.

The rise of suicide and burnout among physicians has created a new disease among healthcare providers we thought only affected soldiers: moral distress syndrome, secondary only to moral injury.

Moral distress syndrome includes depression, PTSD, risk of suicide, divorce, emotional detachment, and the inability to build healthy relationships and empathy.

While veterans can report to a veterans hospital for treatment, physicians may not be able to find treatment or support for fear of losing their license, hospital privileges, or job. Therefore, they're stuck dealing with the issue themselves with only their family or circle of friends for support.

I wrote this book to raise decisive awareness of the problems related to moral distress.

The book is designed to illustrate situations in which a physician is talking to other physicians about the subject of moral distress in a safe space. This book brings together all aspects of moral distress syndrome into a format familiar to physicians grand rounds with a magistral lecture where the audience can ask questions and directly participate with the subject. Readers can get in sync with some of the audience and ask questions as the book progresses.

The book is divided into three parts.

In the first part of the book, the research, data, and a crude number of problems are given: moral distress syndrome, PTSD, burnout, suicide, divorce rates, emotional detachment, legal distress syndrome, physicians leaving medicine, and the feeling of being a hamster in a wheel.

In the second part, I wanted to describe the pain, the emotions, and the symptoms of moral distress by having the main character define some personal experience that gets the reader feeling the depth of it. Therefore, I created stories around the character—their family, love life, divorce, etc.—to show the individual behind the doctor.

In the third part, I focus on society, physician suffering, and the birth of moral distress. This part focuses on the physician's empathy to try to point out his problems, weaknesses, and issues, and find possible solutions to this situation for him and all the other physicians facing the same issues. At the end of the third part, I discuss society's, patients', and physicians' responsibilities, the birth of moral injury, and the American Medical Association's recommendations for dealing with it. We finish with the search for good friends and a safe space, the cornerstones for the healing process.

Structure of the Chapters

At the beginning of each chapter, I outline the points discussed to make it easier to follow the material, just as a speaker outlines the material by summarizing it in the first slide of each topic.

I hope that this structure will help readers focus on the issues quickly throughout the book.

This book is in the format of a business novel, and therefore the characters and situations are fictional but based on real life.

Despite the format of the book as a business novel, the reader can read each chapter separately and be able to understand the main point without the need to follow the story.

What Is Moral Distress?

Moral distress in healthcare was identified by Andrew Jameton (1), who defined it as "knowing what to do in an ethical situation, but not being allowed to do it." Numerous examples of moral distress emerge in everyday clinical practice, starting with the nurse's arena in the last 30 years (2). Only recently, the same concepts were applied to physicians; this is secondary to the fact that most physicians now are hired by corporations and hospitals, and physicians have lost their freedom by joining a structured practice. Corporate rules are now applied, and there is no difference between physicians, nurses, and secretaries. They all must obey rules that makes a big difference for physicians. You cannot ask a physician to sit in an office even if there are no patients to see just because they have a contract but are denied the extra hours on top of the 40 hours a week the physician provides at night or during the weekend. In my previous book, *The Health Care Collapse*, we started recognizing the problem of corporations and its influence on the doctor's ability to practice and their physical reaction to the new situation, including depression and distress secondary to these situations (3).

Moral distress has implications for the satisfaction, recruitment, and retention of healthcare providers and consequences (4) for the delivery of safe and competent quality patient care (5, 6). A key component in recognizing moral distress is a sense of powerlessness. As explained by Savel and Munro (2), these constraints can be internal, such as anxiety or self-doubt about creating conflict, or external, related to power imbalances in the workplace (7). One can distinguish between a moral dilemma, in which there are multiple choices to make, in which the correct path may not be clear, and moral distress, in which the way is clear, but the ability to implement a solution is somehow blocked (8). In 2004, the American Association of Critical-Care Nurses published the four "A"s to rising above moral distress to help nurses to recognize and address moral distress (9). In this document, the four "A"s are presented to help combat the frustrations in these complex situations: ask, affirm, assess, and act. Failure to respond can bring about post-traumatic stress disorder (PTSD) and suicide (8).

Moral Injury

Simon Talbot and Wendy Dean wrote in their article (10) that physicians don't just burn out, they are suffering from a moral injury.

They reported that physicians, like combat soldiers, often face a profound and unrecognized threat to their well-being: moral injury.

> Moral injury is frequently mischaracterized. In combat veterans, it is diagnosed as post-traumatic stress; among physicians, it's portrayed as burnout. But without understanding the critical difference between exhaustion and moral injury, the wounds will never heal, and physicians and patients alike will continue to suffer the consequences (10).

"The term 'moral injury' was first used to describe soldiers' responses to their actions in war. It represents perpetrating, failing to prevent, bearing witness to, or learning about acts that transgress deeply held moral beliefs and expectations." Journalist Diane Silver reported to Talbot and Dean, that it is "a deep soul wound that pierces a person's identity, sense of morality, and relationship to society" (10).

To battle moral distress, one must understand that it exists, understand what it is, and realize that there are structured approaches to help recognize and manage the problem (2, 8).

Why Is It a Syndrome?

Burnout is associated with suicide; they are all connected. These are the same symptoms the soldier experiences after battle or after being deployed. At one time, it was called PTSD. Now it is defined as moral injury or distress since, in many, it is not evident right away and grows in the person with time (11).

Moral distress and moral injury are now the same thing as one brings the other, and with the initial injury, the distress starts and never goes away. It is not just a clinical presentation; it is a constellation of symptoms. Therefore, we can define it as a syndrome because it has many causes, symptoms, and clinical presentations. The following is what I define as moral distress syndrome (12):

1. PTSD
2. Burnout
3. Empathy
4. Emotional detachment
5. Inability to sustain friendships or family duties
6. Divorce
7. Suicide

The presentation can be simple discontent with the job, a complaint of lack of recognition, or can start with a lawsuit. The clinical symptomatology can include the following:

1. Physical: headache, fatigue, insomnia, muscle ache and stiffness, heart palpitations, GI syndrome

2. Mental: inability to concentrate, memory loss, confusion, indecisiveness
3. Emotional: shock, anxiety, nervousness, depression, anger, frustration, worry, fear, irritability, guilt, shame, insecurity
4. Behavioral: hyperactivity, change in eating habits, defensive approach with patients, smoking, drinking, yelling, abusive disorders

Physicians are killing themselves at alarming rates (twice that of active duty military members), signaling something is desperately wrong with the system (10).

Medical licensure applications and renewal applications frequently require answers to broad-based, time-unlimited questions regarding the physician's mental health history without regard to current impairment, and the courts have determined that they are impermissible because the resultant examinations and restrictions constitute discrimination under Title II of the Americans with Disabilities Act (ADA) based on stereotypes (13).

Safe Wellness Program

The problem is that the physician cannot get help. If they look for guidance, they need to report their status, and they can lose their privileges and their board license automatically. There is no safety net, and there is no protection for the physician like a soldier thrown back into the field.

A soldier can rely on the VA system to get treated, and they get disability and other perks; however, the physician is alone in this battle, left abandoned by the hospital, medical organizations, and medical boards.

We need to set a safety net, private psychological support that cannot be reported to anyone, or we will continue to see the suicides increase and physicians burning out of practices. I hope this book will help physicians and corporate hospitals to open their eyes to the issues before it is too late.

References

1. A. Jameton. *Nursing Practice: The Ethical Issues.* Englewood Cliffs, NJ: Prentice-Hall; 1984.
2. R. H. Savel and C. L. Munro. Moral distress and moral courage. *American Journal of Critical Care.* 2015; 24(4):276–278.
3. E. E. Frezza. *The Health Care Collapse.* New York; Routledge; 2018; ISBN # 978-1-138-58110-4.
4. C. Varcoe, J. Storch, and B. M. Pauly. Framing the issues: Moral distress in health care. *Journal of Health and Human Services Administrations*; 2012; 24(1):1–11. https://link.springer.com/article/10.1007/s10730-012-9176-y.
5. C. Westling et al. Perceived ethics dilemmas among pioneer accountable care organizations. *Journal of Healthcare Management*; 2017; 62(1):18; Lippincott Williams & Wilkins Ovid Technologies.
6. M. C. Corley. Nurse moral distress: A proposed theory and research agenda. *Nursing Ethics.* 2002; 9(6):636–650.
7. E. G. Epstein and S. Delgado. Understanding and addressing moral distress. *OJIN: The Online Journal of Issues in Nursing.* 2010; 15(3).
8. A. Gallagher. Moral distress and moral courage in everyday nursing practice. *OJIN: The Online Journal of Issues in Nursing.* 2010; 16(2).
9. American Nurses Association. *Code of Ethics for Nurses with Interpretive Statements.* Published 2015. http://www.nursing-world.org/codeofethics. White paper 2015.
10. S. Talbot and W. Dean. Physicians aren't 'burning out.' They're suffering from moral injury. 2018. https://www.statnews.com/2018/07/26/physicians-not-burning-out-they-are-suffering-moral-injury.
11. J. G. W. S. Wong. Doctors and Stress – The Federation of Medical Societies. *Medical Bulletin*; 2008; 13(6). http://www.fmshk.org/database/articles/03mb1_3.pdf.
12. E. E. Frezza. *Tangled Sutures.* Austin, TX; TMA; 2018. www.texasmedicalassociation.org.

13. AMA 2018 resolution. Memo to: Delegates, Alternate Delegates, Executive Directors, State Medical Associations, National Medical Specialty Societies. AMA; 2018. https://www.ama-assn.org/press-center/press-releases/increasing-awareness-suicide-risks-save-lives.

THE ISSUES FUELING MORAL DISTRESS SYNDROME

1

Chapter 1

Two Old Friends

In this session we will talk about:

- *Getting to know the speaker*
- *Getting to know the audience*
- *Definition of moral distress*

Carlo Bruni was on his way to speak at the NYU Langone Hospital in Brooklyn. His old-time friend Jeremy Spears, now the Department of Surgery chairman, invited him to give the grand round lecture after the morbidity and mortality conference today. Carlo was in his mid-50s, with short hair and no beard and wearing a pair of glasses. He never liked a beard, but never wanted to shave either; he just had to look professional. He was walking from the hotel to the conference room, remembering the time spent with Jeremy. They were chief residents together in Staten Island, where the scent of the beach and the sea mingles with the smell of the New York City dump. It was all by dint of the wind: if it was a good day you could appreciate the seaside scent, but if the wind was blowing from south to north all the trash of New York filled the nostrils.

The two friends always competed to be the best chief resident surgeon. They embarked on problematic cases ranging from liver resection to pancreatic resection with the right amount of fear but with excellent preparation. Carlo was publishing more than Jeremy. He was good at writing papers and book chapters.

He obtained a good fellowship in liver surgery and bariatric surgery while Jeremy applied for a surgical oncology fellowship. Jeremy got the position he sought and then advanced in rank to become chief of surgery. After that, he was named the chair of the department. Carlo followed a similar path, but after achieving his position of chief of surgery nothing went well, and he had to leave his academic institution to defend himself against a long and stressful lawsuit. Now Carlo was working in a private hospital practice, which he completely disliked. But he still had to eat and support his children.

How strange was life? Did everyone believe that Carlo was chairman material and not Jeremy? Life was not as gentle with Carlo, and he knew it. He had to jump through several hoops, and he made it, though with a great deal of suffering and great emotional, family, and financial loss. He arrived at the conference room. It was early, and there were not too many people.

Jeremy came toward him: "Carlo – what a pleasure to see you – we should have gone to dinner last night, but you know my kids needed some help and that would not have worked. Maybe we can do lunch after the conferences." He was in good shape, running outside with his dog every morning, even if it was raining or snowing. He had blond hair and light glasses.

"I am fine," replied Carlo, "the hotel was great and thank you for the bottle of wine you sent to my room."

"Don't mention it. Let me introduce some of the faculty members. This is Dr. Roberts, a surgeon trained in laparoscopy and specializing in robotics. This is Dr. Masai, who is the oncology surgeon. This is Dr. Lopez, the colorectal specialist, and here is Dr. Trincao, the breast specialist." They all shook hands warmly. "Let's go downstairs and get a good cup of coffee before we start; we have a Dunkin Donuts shop and maybe we can get a good bagel like in the old days."

"I miss New York, particularly for the bagels; they have the best bagels ever," said Carlo, and they started laughing.

"A double espresso cappuccino for my friend," said Jeremy, "and a mocha for me."

"How are you doing? How have you been hanging on? You have a lot to tell me. Are you still going to the gym at 4 A.M.?"

Carlo smiled: "Yes, I do; I had to leave for a while when my mind was busy with other life issues, but I went back, and I felt much better."

"How is your wife?"

"My ex," underlined Carlo, "she couldn't cope with the pressure of the situation, and we ended up divorcing, but the children are OK. They did quite well during the process, and they live with her. What about your life?"

"Mine is a full-time job," laughed Jeremy, "Jenny is 16, and you know she is a real 16 with all the teenage psychological issues. Jeremy Jr. is 12 and is doing well. We will see what happens when he becomes a teenager." They laugh again. "And yours?"

"Giovanni is 22 years old and at the University of Delaware and Mario is 19 and at McGill in Canada. They are going strong. They are good children. I thought I lost them, but I found another way to be with them and have a relationship, and it is working well now, probably even better than before."

"Let me get an everything bagel with cream cheese – actually two, right?" said Jeremy. Carlo nodded.

They finished the bagels, and while sipping their coffee, returned to the conference room, which now was crowded. There were residents from surgery, medicine, gynecology, and family practice; medical students; and faculty members from different departments. The topic of the conference must be a hot one, Carlo thought. It is not an everyday conference but one about the moral distress in a physician's life, and he knows about moral distress. Oh yes, God only knows how Carlo was a life expert on the subject.

1.1 Definition of Moral Distress

Jeremy then took the podium. "Good morning everyone. Thank you all for coming this early. I would like to start the day by citing data from a paper I read on Medscape. It has been known

> for more than 150 years that physicians have an increased propensity to die by suicide. It was estimated in 1977 that, on average, the United States loses the equivalent of at least one small medical school or a large medical school class to suicide each year. Exact numbers are not known.

Although it is impossible to estimate with accuracy because of the inaccurate reporting and coding of the cause of death,

> the number most often given is approximately 300 to 400 physicians per year, or perhaps a doctor a day. Of all occupations and professions, the medical profession consistently hovers near the top of professions (1)

with the highest risk of death by suicide. We talked about depression, burnout, and other issues. The road that brings physicians to kill themselves is moral injury and in general, a moral distress situation created by the outside environment. We cannot hide this anymore.

Dear colleagues, residents, and students, it is my honor to present today Dr. Carlo Bruni. We have known each other since residency and I purposely invited him to talk about this challenging subject. The mainstream conference is still hesitant about bringing this subject into the open. Fortunately, or unfortunately, Carlo had extensive personal experience, which marked him for life but he was able to make it, and now he is giving speeches around the country on this subject and how it affects physicians and their families and friends. With the increase in burnout, suicide, and divorce rates, it is important for physicians to recognize moral distress, as the medical society and the state board do not provide help and support in dealing with this issue but rather punish us if we have problems. Therefore, I am happy you are here to hear from Carlo and to ask questions. I reserved the conference room for the entire morning because I expected many questions for our guests. Now without further preamble, please welcome Dr. Bruni."

Reference

1. Louise B. Andrew, and Barry E. Brenner. Physician suicide: Overview, depression in physicians. *Medscape*; 2018. https://emedicine.medscape.com/article/806779-overview.

Suggested Reading

E. E. Frezza. *The Health Care Collapse*. New York; Routledge; 2018; ISBN # 978-1-138-58110-4.

E. E. Frezza. *Tangled Sutures*. Austin, TX; TMA; 2018. www.texasmedicalassociation.org.

E. E. Frezza. *Medical Ethics*. Routledge; 2018. ISBN # 978-1-138-58107-4.

S. Talbot and W. Dean. Physicians aren't 'burning out.' They're suffering from moral injury. 2018. https://www.statnews.com/2018/07/26/physicians-not-burning-out-they-are-suffering-moral-injury.

E. E. Frezza. *The Miserable Doctor*. Sacramento, CA; Cure Your Practice Press; 2019; ISBN # 978-1-7047-7-3056.

Chapter 2

The Grand Round Lecture

In this session we will talk about:

- *Moral distress syndrome*
- *Moral pain*
- *Moral injury*

The audience applauded quietly; they were all worried and afraid to hear what Carlo had to say. They found the idea of physicians suffering from moral distress syndrome disturbing, and in truth, asked themselves if they already had the virus of moral distress.

2.1 Moral Distress Syndrome

"Thank you, Jeremy. It is an honor to be here and to speak in front of all of you. It is a subject that is dear to me since I have seen more and more physicians, residents, and even medical students getting lost in the throes of moral distress syndrome without knowing how to get out. I noticed a significant number across the medical specialties, not just from the department of surgery. That is a good sign because we can all learn something and help other colleagues in need.

We will divide this lecture into different subjects and try to cover the significant factors that lead to moral distress syndrome. To better follow my presentation, before each session I will show you a slide with the points that will be discussed.

My talk will focus on the definition of moral distress syndrome, on the issues of burnout, suicide, lawsuits, divorce rate among physicians, and lost income and retirement funds. I will also recount personal experiences over some years in the past. During the presentation feel free to ask questions."

Then Carlo started with his first slide.

"Moral distress and moral injury are related concepts. One can lead to the other, and both can present in a distress syndrome that once it begins is never resolved. It is not just a symptom; it is a syndrome with many causes, signs, and clinical presentations. The following are all part of moral distress syndrome (1):

1. PTSD (post-traumatic stress disorder)
2. Burnout
3. Empathy
4. Emotional detachment
5. Inability to sustain friendships or family duties
6. Divorce
7. Suicide

The symptoms can vary but most commonly present as headache, fatigue, insomnia, muscle ache and stiffness, and heart palpitations. These usually are followed by inability to concentrate, anxiety, nervousness, depression, and anger. If anger and the depression are not controlled a sense of frustration and general irritability can take over and lead to bad habits including overeating or bulimia, which may be followed by smoking, drinking, yelling, abusive conduct, and other harmful behaviors."

2.2 Moral Pain

"Based on these recurrent problems, on October 9 of the 2018 Interim Meeting of the House of Delegates, the American Medical Association issued a House of Delegates resolution reporting their study of Medical Student, Resident, and Physician Suicide (D-345.984) to determine the most efficient and accurate mechanism to evaluate the actual incidence of medical student, resident, and physician suicide, with recommendations for action (2). The problems have been underevaluated for many years, but now it is time to tackle these issues.

Where does the term moral distress come from? In 1984 Andrew Jameton published the first description of moral distress (3). He defined it as 'knowing what to do in an ethical situation, but not being allowed to do it.' Numerous examples of moral distress emerge in everyday clinical practice (4). These include continued life support, even when it may not be in the best interests of the patient; inadequate communication about end-of-life care among providers, patients, and families; inappropriate use of healthcare resources; inadequate staffing; and false hope given to patients and families. A key component in recognizing moral distress is a sense of powerlessness (5).

The definition of moral distress took a left curve in the last 20 years.

In 2004, the American Association of Critical-Care Nurses published *The 4As to Rising Above Moral Distress* to help clinicians recognize and address moral distress (6).

The 4As to help survive the frustrations are: ask, affirm, assess, and act. Moral distress occurs at work when an employee feels unable to move by his or her values or obligations. Seventy-seven percent of Veterans Affairs (VA) employees experience moral distress. Common causes in healthcare settings include difficulty speaking up, poor team communications and teamwork, concerns about patient safety, uncertainty about which practices are ethical, and conflicts of values in end-of-life decision making. Moral distress can decrease job satisfaction, morale, and job retention. These issues can directly affect patient safety and quality of care (7).

The distress of not being able to take the right course of action was still the focus in the definition of moral distress, which: 'occurs when one [believes one] knows the right thing to do, but institutional or other constraints make it difficult to pursue the desired course of action' (8).

These constraints can be internal, such as anxiety or self-doubt about creating conflict, or external, related to power imbalances in the workplace (9). One can distinguish between a moral dilemma, in which there are multiple choices to make, and the correct path may not be clear, and moral distress, in which the road is clear, but the ability to implement a solution is somehow blocked (10).

Moral distress in healthcare has been identified as a growing concern and a focus of research in nursing and healthcare for almost three decades. Researchers and theorists have argued that moral distress has both short- and long-term consequences. Moral distress has implications for satisfaction, recruitment, and retention of providers and implications for the delivery of safe and competent quality patient care. In over a decade of research on ethical practice, registered nurses and other healthcare practitioners have repeatedly identified moral distress as a concern and called for action. However, research and activity on moral distress have been constrained by a lack of conceptual clarity and intellectual confusion as to the meaning and underpinnings of moral pain (11)."

2.3 Moral Injury

"Simon Talbot and Wendy Dean wrote (12) that physicians don't just burn out. They reported that physicians, like combat soldiers, often face a profound and unrecognized threat to their well-being: moral injury.

Moral injury is frequently mischaracterized. In combat veterans, it is diagnosed as post-traumatic stress disorder (PTSD); among physicians, it's portrayed as burnout. But without understanding the critical difference between exhaustion and moral injury, the wounds will never heal, and physicians and patients alike will continue to suffer the consequences.

The term 'moral injury' was first used to describe soldiers' responses to their actions in war. It represents "perpetrating, failing to prevent, bearing witness to, or learning about acts that transgress deeply held moral beliefs and expectations." Journalist Diane Silver reported it to Talbot and Dean as 'a deep soul wound that pierces a person's identity, sense of morality, and relationship to society' (12).

Talbot and Dean concluded that to ensure that compassionate, engaged, highly skilled physicians are leading patient care, executives in the healthcare system must recognize and then acknowledge that this is not purely physician burnout. Physicians are dying by suicide at alarming rates (twice that of active duty military members), signaling something is desperately wrong with the system (12)."

2.4 Moral Distress

"Moral distress is accentuated when things do not go well. Sometimes we know what we want to do but are unable to execute our desired action plan. Perhaps it's because we're providing care we deem inappropriate. Or maybe we believe families are being given false hope. These pangs we feel needn't be patient related, however: whenever our moral compass is being spun against our will, we feel wounded. We go home feeling a terrible combination of anger, fear, confusion, and powerlessness. To battle moral distress, one must understand that it exists, understand what it is, and realize that there are structured approaches to help recognize and manage the problem" (8). Carlo continues his presentation.

"Healthcare is based on taking care of patients, and only the physician can do this to the fullest extent. Now, however, many factors play a role, and the physician is losing ground. The major problem I see is that physicians have no significant recognition or rewards, neither monetary, as we are not making the same salary as 20 years ago, nor emotional, as legislation has relegated us to the role of secretaries doing administrative office work, and we are made to spend more time on paperwork than on patient care. But we are more than that, much more!

We are always in the front line like soldiers ready to take the bullets while the others are ready to go home, and we are developing PTSD (13)! We have no recognition or reward and more duty and legislation, which makes us spend more time on paperwork than on patients care."

References

1. E. E. Frezza. *Tangled Sutures*. Austin, TX; TMA; 2018. www.tex asmedicalassociation.org.
2. ama-assn.org. Report 21 of the Board of Trustees (A-19). Augmented Intelligence (AI) in Health Care. 2019. https://www .ama-assn.org/system/files/2019-04/a19-702.pdf.
3. A. Jameton. *Nursing Practice: The Ethical Issues*. Englewood Cliffs, NJ; Prentice-Hall; 1984.
4. M. C. Corley. Nurse moral distress: A proposed theory and research agenda. *Nursing Ethics*. 2002; 9(6):636–650.

5. R. H. Savel and C. L. Munro. Moral distress, moral courage: Critical care nursing. *American Journal of Critical Care*; 2015; 24(4):276–278. http://ajcc.aacnjournals.org/content/24/4/276. doi: 10.4037/ajcc2015738.

6. American Nurses Association. *Code of Ethics for Nurses with Interpretive Statements*; 2015. http://www.nursingworld.org/codeofethics.

7. Moral distress initiative: Organizational excellence. https://www.va.gov/HEALTHCAREEXCELLENCE/about/organization/examples/moral-distress.

8. Moral distress: Healthy debate. November 10, 2018. https://healthydebate.ca/opinions/moral_distress.

9. E. G. Epstein and S. Delgado. Understanding and addressing moral distress. *OJIN: The Online Journal of Issues in Nursing*. 2010; 15(3). Moral distress: Healthy debate. https://healthydebate.ca/opinions/moral_distress.

10. A. Gallagher. Moral distress and moral courage in everyday nursing practice. *OJIN: The Online Journal of Issues in Nursing*. 2010; 16(2).

11. B. M. Pauly, C. Varcoe, and J. Storch. Framing the issues: Moral distress in health care. *HEC Forum*; 2012; 24(1):1–11. https://link.springer.com/article/10.1007%2Fs10730-012-9176-y.

12. S. Talbot and W. Dean. Physicians aren't 'burning out.' They're suffering from moral injury. 2018. https://www.statnews.com/2018/07/26/physicians-not-burning-out-they-are-suffering-moral-injury.

13. E. E. Frezza. *The Miserable Doctor*. Sacramento, CA; Cure Your Practice Press; 2019; ISBN # 978-1-7047-7-3056.

Chapter 3

Litigation Syndrome

In this session we will talk about:

- *Litigation syndrome*
- *Burnout and suicide*
- *Emotional detachment*

3.1 Definition and Symptoms of Litigation Syndrome

In a Texas Medical Association publication we defined litigation syndrome as the condition affecting physicians who are experiencing a lawsuit and reported its symptoms (1):

1. Physical: Headache, fatigue, insomnia, muscle ache and stiffness, heart palpitation, gastrointestinal disorders
2. Mental: Inability to concentrate, memory loss, confusion, indecisiveness
3. Emotional: Shock, anxiety, nervousness, depression, anger, frustration, worry, fear, irritability, guilt, shame, insecurity
4. Behavioral: Hyperactivity, change in eating habits, defensive approach with patients, smoking, drinking, yelling, abusive behavior

These are symptoms secondary to stress, which add to the practical, patient, hospital, or family issues (2). Stress may adversely affect not only the individual doctor but also his or her family life, marriage, and social life. At the same time, since the pressure of being a physician today is already high, malpractice litigation can bring the physician over the edge. Stress is associated with burnout (3, 4) and moral injury!

3.2 Burnout and Suicide

Burnout is associated with suicides. These are the same symptoms soldiers experience after deployment or a battle. At one time it was called PTSD (post-traumatic stress disorder). Now it is defined as moral injury or moral distress since, in many, it is not evident right away and develops over the years (5). As reported by Frezza in *Medical Ethics* (6), these are the data for high-risk suicide groups:

- Depression among medical residents rises to 30%
- Litigations and lawsuits create more imbalance and increase the risk above 50%
- Male physicians have a 50–70% higher risk than the general population
- Female physicians have a 400% increased risk than the average population
- Burnout is secondary to high demand from patients and the health system

A person who can effectively utilize emotional detachment can set apparent boundaries. Be it in social situations, during family strife, or in their professional discernment, these people earn great respect for their ability to remain calm and make clear decisions, all the while respecting the emotions of others. For the majority of people, emotional detachment is a far cry from reality. Choosing not to engage when emotions run high seems impossible for most people. Unfortunately, the news media, entertainment sources, politicians, and even religious leaders can feed this disempowering lie. Done right, emotional detachment includes empathy. Without empathy, emotional detachment would be malignant. There is a common myth that compassion requires vulnerability. It is only through honest emotional detachment that one can be of service with compassion.

This is the balance a doctor strives for every day. Whether we must give a patient bad news, or we are helping them come to an informed decision from an emotionally charged place, we must first empathize, and then we must detach. A doctor must learn emotional detachment, and he or she must own it completely. Any doctor can find themselves in the face of shocking trauma at most any time; it's one of the characteristics of the profession. This is why doctors often have an air of authority and are often seen as wise (3, 7).

3.3 Emotional Detachment

Emotional detachment in empathy allows one space to rationally choose their responses without being drawn into an overwhelming state or being manipulated. Emotional boundary management is a useful and common tool. Whether responding to an overwrought patient or an overwhelmed peer, control of emotional boundaries is crucial to maintaining one's integrity, dignity, and choice capacity.

There is almost a mystique around a self-possessed, emotionally detached person. The skill is so rare as to inspire awe in many. The simple act (once learned) of deciding to step aside from current drama is compelling. Anyone can learn it, but few realize this (5, 7).

"Innocent until proven guilty" is profoundly flawed. In reality, it feels like "guilty until proven innocent"! That's what it feels like. Everyone looks at the physician who is being sued like they are a criminal. It doesn't even matter if the charge isn't all that damning (8, 9).

References

1. E. E. Frezza. *Tangled Sutures*. Austin, TX; TMA; 2018. www.tex asmedicalassociation.org.
2. C. Varcoe, J. Storch, and B. M. Pauly. Framing the issues: Moral distress in health care. *Journal of Health and Human Services Administrations*. 2012. https://link.springer.com/article/10.1007/s10730-12-9176-y.
3. J. G. W. S. Wong. Doctors and stress – The Federation of Medical Societies. *Medical Bulletin*; 2008; 13(6). http://www.fmshk.org/database/articles/03mb1_3.pdf
4. E. E. Frezza. *The Miserable Doctor*. Sacramento, CA; Cure Your Practice Press; 2019; ISBN # 978-1-7047-7-3056.
5. S. Talbot and W. Dean. Physicians aren't 'burning out.' They're suffering from moral injury. 2018. https://www.statnews.com/2018/07/26/physicians-not-burning-out-they-are-suffering-moral-injury.
6. E. E. Frezza. *Medical Ethics*. New York; Routledge; 2018; ISBN # 978-1-138-58107-4.
7. R. H. Savel and C. L. Munro. Moral distress and moral courage. *American Journal of Critical Care*. 2015; 24(4):276–278.
8. E. G. Epstein and S. Delgado. Understanding and addressing moral distress. *OJIN: The Online Journal of Issues in Nursing*. 2010; 15(3).
9. B. M. Pauly, C. Varcoe, and J. Storch. Framing the issues: Moral distress in health care. *HEC Forum*; 2012; 24(1):1–11. https://link.springer.com/article/10.1007%2Fs10730-12-9176-y.

Suggested Reading

E. E. Frezza. *The Health Care Collapse*. New York; Routledge; 2018; ISBN # 978-1-138-58110-4.
M. C. Corley. Nurse moral distress: A proposed theory and research agenda. *Nursing Ethics*. 2002; 9(6):636–650.

A. Gallagher. Moral distress and moral courage in everyday nursing practice. *OJIN: The Online Journal of Issues in Nursing.* 2010; 16(2).

American Nurses Association. *Code of Ethics for Nurses with Interpretive Statements.* 2015. http://www.nursingworld.org/codeofethics.

E. L. Vliet. Physician suicide rates have climbed since Obamacare passed. *Physician News Digest,* 2015. https://physiciansnews.com/2015/05/19/physician-suicide-rates-have-climbed-since-obamacare-passed/.

L. B. Andrew. Physician suicide. *Medscape.* 2018. https://emedicine.medscape.com/article/806779-overview.

E. Elizabeth. Famous holistic doctor & wife allegedly jump to death off Manhattan Office Highrise – Leave Typed Suicide Notes. 2017. https://www.healthnutnews.com/famous-holistic-doctor-wife-allegedly-jump-to-death.

AMA 2018 resolution. Report 21 of the Board of Trustees (A-19). Augmented Intelligence (AI) in Health Care. 2018. https://www.ama-assn.org/press-center/press-releases/increasing-awareness-suicide-risks-save-lives.

Physician suicide: Overview, depression in physicians. http://emedicine.medscape.com/article/806779-overview.

Chapter 4

Burnout

In this session we will talk about:

- *Causes of burnout*
- *The side effects of burnout*
- *Suicide and PTSD*
- *Depression syndrome even in medical students*
- *Must be healthy to get licensure*

4.1 Causes of Burnout

The audience was completely silent; not even the sound of breathing of the people in the front row could be heard. Carlo took a deep breath and continued.

"Post-traumatic stress disorder (PTSD) brings distress and distress brings burnout! Burnout is a significant problem in the United States and is reaching a rate of 70% among physicians. Burnout is characterized by emotional exhaustion and fatigue and possibly a loss of a sense of personal accomplishment, and has significant consequences for both individual providers and the healthcare organization."

4.2 Side Effects of Burnout

"Interestingly, burnout is recognized by many companies and industries but not in healthcare. It is very difficult for a physician to admit burnout, depression, and other symptomatology because of possible repercussions: if you talk to someone it will be reported to the board and your license may be restricted or suspended.

Physical complications of increased stress are well known. These include insomnia, gastrointestinal disturbance, tension headaches, hypertension, fatigue, lowered immunity, menstrual irregularities, and sexual dysfunction. As noted previously in this book, stress may adversely affect not only the individual doctor but also his or her family life, marriage, and social life. Furthermore, stress is associated with burnout (1)."

4.3 Suicide and PTSD

"Physicians, in general, have a higher rate of suicide than members of other professional groups and the public in general. According to an article by Elizabeth Lee Vliet in the *Physician Digest*, women physicians' suicide rates are reported to be up to 400% higher than those of women in other professions (2). Male physicians' rates are 50% to 70% higher than in the general population.

Physicians have a lower mortality risk from cancer and heart disease relative to the general population (presumably related to knowledge of self-care and early diagnosis), but they have a significantly higher risk of dying by suicide. Suicide is the most common cause of death among medical students as well (3).

It has been known for more than 150 years that physicians have an increased propensity to die by suicide. It was estimated in 1977 that on average the United States loses approximately 300–400 physicians/year, one doctor each day (4). The medical profession is consistently near the top of occupations with the highest risk of death by suicide.

Burnout is one of the causes of a decrease in quality care and patient satisfaction but also affects the private life of the physician, which can end in drug addiction and increase the risk of suicide. On the professional side, it can increase medical errors and malpractice risk.

The physician provides care for people, but there are few provisions in the healthcare system to care for the physician. Most physicians report the cause of burnout is secondary to work overload, insufficient rewards, unfair treatment by the hospital healthcare system, and breakdown in communication between them and healthcare administrators. There is a pervasive conflict of values between healthcare facilities and the physician, with a push toward producing more, with the risk of a decrease in quality. The physician is overwhelmed by bureaucratic tasks that take away from valuable patient care time and increase the risk of medical malpractice as well. Physicians are also concerned that they do not have enough time for continuous medical education while spending more time documenting the electronic medical record. The latter system is built by nonphysicians for use by physicians and often does not align with clinical practice; therefore, the documentation is lengthy and elaborated while often missing essential information.

According to Talbot and Dean, burnout is a constellation of symptoms that include exhaustion, cynicism, and decreased productivity. More than half of physicians report at least one of these. But the concept of burnout resonates poorly with physicians: it suggests a failure of resourcefulness and resilience, traits that most physicians have finely honed during decades of intense training and demanding work. Even at the Mayo Clinic, which has been tracking, investigating, and addressing burnout for more than a decade, one-third of physicians report symptoms of burnout (5).

Physicians are not part of the medical decision-making and strategic choices in a hospital and do not participate in crucial meetings to discuss a new algorithm for treating patients; they therefore grow frustrated.

In a situation in which someone else in the department faces serious censure, physicians feel they are the second victims, as I can relate from personal experience. At one time I was working in an organization where the president went to jail and my boss died by suicide. Everyone who had had a professional relationship with these individuals became the 'second victim' and was pushed out of the hospital. Having experienced this, it's my firm belief that it should never happen to anyone. Physicians lost control of their medical practice, and they feel that they are not rewarded. There is a sense of unfairness regarding doing more work for less, and they perceive a conflict between the profit motive and the quality of care.

Most organizations hire physicians based on a 40-hour work week, but in actuality physicians double those hours. Their extra hours are not recognized, and therefore their hourly rate becomes more similar to that for nurses."

4.4 Depression Symptoms Even in Medical Students

"Physicians have a higher likelihood of depression relative to the general population (6), with a significantly higher risk of dying secondary to depression and suicide. Depression is at least as common in the medical profession as for the general population, affecting an estimated 12% of men and up to 19.5% of women.

Depression is even more prevalent in medical students and residents, with 15–30% screening positive for depressive symptoms (7). This is common also in other countries such as Finland, Norway, Australia, Singapore, China, Taiwan, and Sri Lanka.

Litigation-related stress can precipitate depression and, occasionally, suicide. Some physicians have completed suicide on a first receipt of malpractice claims, after judgments against them in court, or after financially motivated settlements foisted upon them by a malpractice insurer solely to cut the insurer's losses. Any agreement in a malpractice case is by law reported to the National Practitioner Data Bank, which is yet another source of distress and stigma that can contribute to depression (8).

Physicians who have reported depressive symptoms (even those for which they are receiving active treatment) to their licensing boards, potential employers, hospitals, and other credentialing agencies have experienced a range of negative consequences, including loss of their medical privacy and autonomy, repetitive and intrusive examinations, licensure restrictions, discriminatory employment decisions, practice restrictions, hospital privilege limitations, and increased supervision (8)."

There was a question from the audience: "Is there anything our medical societies are doing? I am Dr. Metha, by the way, from Obstetrics and Gynecology."

"No indeed," continued Carlo. "Because of the stigma associated with depression, self-reporting likely underestimates the prevalence of the disease in medical populations. It is also a leading risk factor for myocardial infarction in men in general and in physicians, and it may play a role in immune suppression, thus increasing the risk of many infectious diseases and cancer."

4.5 Must Be Healthy to Get Licensures

"The physician feels an obligation to appear healthy, perhaps as evidence of their ability to heal others. The concerned colleague or partner may say nothing while wondering privately if the colleague has become impaired.

Medical licensure applications and renewal applications frequently require answers to broad-based, time-unlimited questions regarding the physician's mental health history without regard to current impairment. The courts have determined that they are impermissible and unconstitutional because the resultant examinations and restrictions constitute discrimination under Title II of the Americans with Disabilities Act (ADA) based on stereotypes (8).

Physicians also fear losing hospital privileges if treatment for depression is disclosed. Hospital administrators increasingly use mandated psychiatric treatment as a bullying tactic to remove independent-thinking, patient-focused physicians from hospital staff.

Because many states require reporting by other licensed physicians of a physician who may be suffering from a potentially impairing condition, physicians can be reluctant to seek treatment from colleagues. They don't want to utilize their insurance coverage or even use their own names when seeking treatment. A physician whose thought processes are clouded by depression and the anticipated consequences of seeking treatment for it may honestly believe that self-treatment is the only safe option (8)."

References

1. J. G. W. S Wong. Doctors and stress. *Medical Bulletin*; 2008. http://www.fmshk.org/database/articles/03mb1_3.pdf.
2. E. L. Vliet. Physician suicide rates have climbed since Obamacare passed. *Physician News Digest*; 2019. https://physiciansnews.com/2015/05/19/physician-suicide-rates-have-climbed-since-obamacare-passed/.
3. L. B. Andrew. Physician suicide. *Medscape*. 2018. https://emedicine.medscape.com/article/806779-overview.
4. E. Elizabeth. Famous holistic doctor and wife allegedly jump to death off Manhattan office highrise – leave typed suicide notes. 2017. https://www.healthnutnews.com/famous-holistic-doctor-wife-allegedly-jump-to-death.

5. S. Talbot and W. Dean. Physicians aren't 'burning out.' They're suffering from moral injury. 2018. https://www.statnews.com/2018/07/26/physicians-not-burning-out-they-are-suffering-moral-injury.

6. Why do doctors commit suicide? *The Indian Sun*; 2018. https://www.theindiansun.com.au/2018/10/17/doctors-commit-suicide/.

7. S. Reddy. Difficult patient vs difficult doctor. 2018. https://bioethicsdiscussion.blogspot.com/2018/01/difficult-patient-vs-difficult-doctor.html.

8. Physician suicide: Overview, depression in physicians. https://emedicine.medscape.com/article/806779-overview.

Suggested Reading

A. Jameton. *Nursing Practice: The Ethical Issues.* Englewood Cliffs, NJ; Prentice-Hall; 1984.

R. H. Savel and C. L. Munro. Moral distress and moral courage. *American Journal of Critical Care.* 2015; 24(4):276–278.

E. E. Frezza. *The Health Care Collapse.* New York; Routledge; 2018; ISBN # 978-1-138-58110-4.

C. Varcoe, J. Storch, and B. M. Pauly. Framing the issues: Moral distress in health care. *Journal of Health and Human Services Administrations.* 2012. https://link.springer.com/article/10.1007/s10730-12-9176-y.

M. C. Corley. Nurse moral distress: A proposed theory and research agenda. *Nursing Ethics.* 2002; 9(6):636–650.

E. G. Epstein and S. Delgado. Understanding and addressing moral distress. *OJIN: The Online Journal of Issues in Nursing.* 2010; 15(3).

A. Gallagher. Moral distress and moral courage in everyday nursing practice. *OJIN: The Online Journal of Issues in Nursing.* 2010; 16(2).

American Nurses Association. *Code of Ethics for Nurses with Interpretive Statements.* 2015. http://www.nursingworld.org/codeofethics.

E. E. Frezza. *Tangled Sutures.* Austin, TX; TMA; 2018. www.texasmedicalassociation.org.

E. E. Frezza. *Medical Ethics.* New York; Routledge; 2018; ISBN # 978-1-138-58107-4.

E. E. Frezza. *The Miserable Doctor.* Sacramento, CA; Cure Your Practice Press; 2019; ISBN # 978-1-7047-7-3056.

AMA 2018 resolution. Report 21 of the Board of Trustees (A-19). Augmented Intelligence (AI) in Health Care. 2018. https://www .ama-assn.org/press-center/press-releases/increasing-awareness -suicide-risks-save-lives.

Chapter 5

Suicide: From Medical Student, to Resident, to Clinician

In this session we will talk about:

- *Risk of suicide in physicians*
- *Stress factors and side effects*
- *Suicide in the USA*
- *Lack of policies*

5.1 Risk of Suicide in Physicians

"It has been known for more than 150 years that physicians have an increased propensity to die by suicide. It was estimated in 1977 that, on average, the United States loses to suicide the equivalent of approximately 300–400 physicians/year, a doctor each day. The medical profession is consistently near the top of occupations with the highest risk of death by suicide (1)."

The audience all agree and nod. Carlo resumed: "Perhaps even more alarming is that, after accidents, suicide is the most common cause of death among medical students" (2).

A member of the audience responded: "This data is very worrisome. I am Jane, a third-year medical student. I am just starting my clinical rotation, and now I don't know what to think. What do you think all of this is due to?"

"Jane," said Carlo, "this is a problem. There are good reasons for starting prevention work in medical school. Medical students are our future doctors."

Medical education is, in itself, a stressful process (3). A previous study found elevated depression, anxiety, and stress in local medical students. Students' mental health affects their academic success, social life, and the quality of service they provide to the community as future doctors. Moreover, their mental distress may influence the way they perceive mental health and help-seeking in the care of their prospective patients. A 2003 Royal College of Psychiatrists Report (4) outlined a fundamental responsibility of medical schools to ensure that their graduates are (a) aware of their personal and professional limitations; (b) willing to seek help when necessary, and (c) mindful of the importance of their own health, including mental health, and its impact on their ability to practice as a doctor (5).

5.2 Stress Factors and Side Effects

"You know, Jane," continued Carlo, "in every population, suicide is almost invariably the result of untreated or inadequately treated depression or other mental illness that may or may not include substance or alcohol abuse, coupled with knowledge of and access to lethal means.

Depression is at least as common in the medical profession as in the general population, affecting an estimated 12% of males and up to 19.5% of females. Depression is even more common in medical students and residents, with 15–30% screening positive for depressive symptoms. This is not an isolated North American phenomenon. Studies from Finland, Norway, Australia, Singapore, China, Taiwan, Sri Lanka, and others have shown an increased prevalence of anxiety, depression, and suicidality among students and practitioners of medicine (6).

As you can see in my next slide, stress factors that affect physicians, residents, and medical students are multiple:

- Frustration
- Inner tension
- Difficulty concentrating
- Insomnia
- Family and social withdrawal
- Irritability
- Loss of interest
- Fatigue
- Decreased sex drive
- Gastrointestinal symptoms
- Suicidal ideation

The inability to cope successfully may lead to maladaptive behavioral patterns such as:

- Aloofness
- Irritability
- Disruptive behaviors
- Increased use of alcohol or drugs
- Increased risk of unethical behaviors"

5.3 Suicide in the USA

"The worst consequence of all, though, is suicide, which has been consistently on the rise in the medical profession since the early 2000s and doubling almost every year. Physicians, in general, have a higher rate of suicide than other professional groups and the public in general. Women physicians' suicide rates are reported to be up to 400% higher than those of women in other professions. Male physicians' rates are 50–70% higher (7). The following are some statistics on suicide in the USA:

- It is the seventh leading cause of death in US men
- It is the fifth leading cause of death in US women
- It is the third leading cause of death in the USA among young adults aged 15–24
- It is most prevalent in the elderly and adolescents
- The highest rate is in men over 85 years of age
- Physician health experts say as many as 400 US physicians take their lives each year
- Major depressive disorder (MDD) affects 13–17% of Americans every year
- The rate of MDD in physicians is similar to that of the general population: 13% of male physicians and 20% of female physicians
- One-third of medical residents have a diagnosable MDD during residency
- 30% of physicians show MDD one year after graduation
- MDD is a risk factor for suicide
- Physicians who attempt suicide are much more likely to complete it than non-physicians
- The rate of suicide in male physicians is 70% higher, and the rate in female physicians is 400% higher than in the general population"

5.4 Lack of Policies

Someone raised his hand. "I am Dr. Smith, Chair of Medicine. How can what is going on with our population of physicians be possible? Why?"

Carlo explained: "Demands on physicians have changed and navigating healthcare has become more complex and challenging. Proper action needs to be taken to protect physician and trainee wellness.

Major health organizations have not yet made policy changes despite the evident crises that present a problem with physician suicide. One million Americans are made aware that some of their doctors kill themselves every year.

Between 2017 and 2020, more than 40% of fellow physicians and residents have faced symptoms of anxiety or depression. Residents have felt isolated without ways to seek mental health resources. Many physicians fear the negative consequences and stigma surrounding the admission of mental health diagnoses (8).

Unfortunately, this is concerning not only with regard to practicing physicians. On the Accreditation Council for Graduate Medical Education (ACGME) website there is an entire page dedicated to suicide among medical residents. However, despite adequate information regarding physician suicide and physician wellness, there are no resources that can translate into the everyday lives of physicians, especially trainees (9)."

"Is that not related to internal medicine, right?" rebutted Dr. Smith.

"These are for all, including your specialty," continued Carlo. "'Nine of 10 doctors discourage others from joining the profession, and 300 physicians commit suicide every year,' according to the internist Dr. Daniela Drake. 'Since 1858, suicide among doctors has been increasing exponentially.' A family physician, Dr. Pamela Wible, points out that suicide is the 'second-leading cause of death for residents,'and according to Dr. Nathaniel P. Morris, resident physician in psychiatry at Stanford University School of Medicine, it is the leading cause for male residents (9)."

References

1. L. B. Andrew. Physician suicide: Overview, depression in physicians. *Medscape*; 2018. https://emedicine.medscape.com/article/806779-overview.
2. Why do doctors commit suicide? *The Indian Sun*; 2018. https://www.theindiansun.com.au/2018/10/17/doctors-commit-suicide/.
3. S. Reddy. Difficult patient vs difficult doctor. 2018. https://bioethicsdiscussion.blogspot.com/2018/01/difficult-patient-vs-difficult-doctor.html.
4. S. Kumar. Burnout in psychiatrists. *World Psychiatry*; 2007; 6(3):186–189. https://www.ncbi.nlm.nih.gov/pmc/articles/PMC2175073/.
5. J. G. W. S. Wong. Doctors and stress. The Federation of Medical Societies. *Medical Bulletin*; 2008; 13(6). http://www.fmshk.org/database/articles/03mb1_3.pdf.
6. L. B. Andrew. Physician suicide: Overview, depression in physicians. *Medscape*; 2018. https://emedicine.medscape.com/article/806779-overview.
7. E. L. Vliet. Physician suicide rates have climbed since Obamacare passed. *Physician News Digest*; 2019. https://physiciansnews.com/2015/05/19/physician-suicide-rates-have-climbed-since.
8. K. J. Kelleher and J. Stevens. Evolution of child mental health services in primary care. *Academic Pediatrics*; 2009; 9(1):7–14. doi: 10.1016/j.acap.2008.11.008.
9. E. E. Frezza. *Tangled Sutures*. Austin, TX; TMA; 2018. www.texasmedicalassociation.org.

Suggested Reading

E. E. Frezza. *Medical Ethics*. New York; Routledge; 2018; ISBN # 978-1-138-58107-4.

E. E. Frezza. *The Miserable Doctor*. Sacramento, CA; Cure Your Practice Press; 2019; ISBN # 978-1-7047-7-3056.

E. E. Frezza. *The Health Care Collapse*. New York; Routledge; 2018; ISBN # 978-1-138-58110-4.

Chapter 6

Why Have Physicians Suffered a Lack of Recognition?

In this session we will talk about:

■ *Stressful profession*
■ *Lack of satisfaction*
■ *Lack of respect toward physicians*
■ *Lack of recognition*
■ *Physicians are at risk*
■ *Fear of losing the license*

6.1 Stressful Profession

"I am Dr. Raw, chair of family practice. So why are physicians so much affected?"

Carlo took a deep breath and answered:

"The medical profession is generally perceived as a very stressful occupation. Although some stressors in healthcare settings are inevitable and invariable, such as dealing with incurable patients and their deaths, there are some variable workplace stressors that represent a risk for medical professionals: work organization, financial issues, administration, interference with family and social life, relationships with colleagues and patients, and work demand (long working hours, workload, and pressure). The most common stressors are:

- Demands of the profession and patients
- Lack of sleep
- Poor eating habits and level of fitness
- Exposure to illness, tragedy, and death
- Oversight
- Access to medications
- Burnout
- Implicit discouragement by the medical profession of help-seeking in its members
- Discrimination in medical licensing, hospital privileges, health insurance, professional liability insurance, and professional advancement often directed toward physicians with psychiatric illnesses
- Lack of a regular source of healthcare by 35% of physicians"

6.2 Lack of Satisfaction

"I am Mr. Diehl, CEO of the hospital. So is it the lack of patient appreciation or the lack of satisfaction? It seems the doctors have everything they need."

"It is the physician experience, the experience of being treated similarly to the front desk people, but they have more responsibilities that are not recognized," replied Carlo. "Doctors have always been at higher risk of suicide than other professions for several reasons:

- Pressures of responsibility to save lives
- Fear of making mistakes that can result in a lawsuit

- Fear of losing the medical license
- Long hours, time away from home, no rest
- High incidence of depression and alcohol or substance abuse

As you can see in my next slide, the following are behaviors of physicians caused by their demoralized feelings:

- Mourning
- Systemic anxiety
- Guilt and blame
- Anger and rage at the deceased patient
- Business as usual
- Broken contract
- A sense of betrayal and abandonment
- Severed relationships
- An interruption in healthcare delivery
- Anger
- Burden of trust issues for the next physician"

6.3 Lack of Recognition

"One way to solve some of the problems would be to increase the respect accorded physicians: for the greater number of hours worked, for the quality of work, for the job in the community. Monetary and public awards need to be in place to honor hard-working physicians in clinical practice. To quote Mark Twain, 'I can live for two months on a good compliment.'

More than a century later this is still true; any organizational change initiative would be uncertain, but when change is successful, it is essential to recognize the effort of the team and the individuals involved and reward them.

Thank the physician in a personal way, both privately and in public, not just via an email, letter, or note. More recognition can encourage the person to achieve further goals as well as promote individual growth. Most crucial is timeliness; one should not wait a month before thanking people for their achievements on your behalf."

"I am Marla, a third-year resident in surgery. What possible benefit will dying have anyhow?"

"You are right, Marla," said Carlo, "not much benefit at all. Look at my next slides for the answer. In the first slide I summarize the possible reasons why a person may want to die:

- Fulfill the desire to die
- Escape from an intolerable situation
- Escape from a terrible state of mind
- Escape from intractable pain
- Avoid loss of control
- Make people understand how desperate they were feeling (1)"

6.4 Physicians Are at Risk

"In the next slide, I summarize the factors that can play a role and place the physician at even greater risk:

- Age (adolescent/elderly)
- Male gender
- Unmarried
- Caucasian
- Stigma
- Access to medications or firearms
- Impulsive behavior
- Family history of suicide
- Mental disorders or substance abuse
- Family violence including physical and sexual abuse

- Feelings of hopelessness
- Cultural and religious beliefs

You need to remember that suicidal ideation is strongly related to:

- Burnout
- Emotional exhaustion
- Depersonalization
- Low personal accomplishment

Perceived major medical error in the previous three months, lawsuits, and malpractice claims are major factors in the increase of burnout and suicide. But what is the real problem for the doctors?"

Jeremy raised his hand: "No one talks about suicide – especially in the medical community."

"Exactly right, no one, and the people who need help are left alone to deal with that," answered Carlo.

6.5 Fear of Losing the License

"The problem is that physicians cannot seek help. If they look for guidance, they need to report their status, and can automatically lose their privileges and their board license. There is no safety net and no protection for the physician who has lost faith in themselves; you leave them back in the field and close the door.

However, because of the stigma associated with depression, self-reporting likely underestimates the prevalence of the disease in medical populations. It is also a leading risk factor for myocardial infarction in male physicians, and it may play a role in immune suppression, thus increasing the risk of many infectious diseases and cancer (2, 3).

Physicians also fear losing hospital privileges if treatment for depression is disclosed. As noted in a previous chapter, hospital administrators increasingly use mandated psychiatric treatment as a bullying tactic to remove independent-thinking, patient-focused physicians from hospital staff (4).

Because many states require reporting by other licensed physicians of a physician who may be suffering from a potentially impairing condition, physicians can be reluctant to seek treatment from colleagues, or from utilizing their insurance coverage, or even from using their own names when seeking treatment. A physician whose thought processes are clouded by depression and the likely consequences of seeking treatment for it may honestly believe that self-treatment is the only safe option (5)."

References

1. Teen suicide prevention key: Webinar suicidal R&PT. 2020. https://www.keystosaferschools.com/suicidal-recognition-prev ention-online-training/suicide-prevent-webinar/teen-suicide-prevention-key.
2. L. B. Andrew. Physician suicide: Overview, depression in physicians. 2018. http://emedicine.medscape.com/article/806779-overview.
3. S. Talbot and W. Dean. Physicians aren't 'burning out.' They're suffering from moral injury. *Stat News*; 2018. https://www.sta tnews.com/2018/07/26/physicians-not-burning-out-they-are-suf fering-moral-injury.
4. L. B. Andrew. Physician suicide. *Medscape*. 2018. https://em edicine.medscape.com/article/806779-overview.
5. E. L. Vliet. Physician suicide rates have climbed since obamacare passed. *Physician News Digest*; 2015. https://physiciansne ws.com/2015/05/19/physician-suicide-rates-have-climbed-since-obamacare-passed/.

Suggested Reading

E. E. Frezza. *The Health Care Collapse*. New York; Routledge; 2018; ISBN # 978-1-138-58110-4.

C. Varcoe, J. Storch, and B. M. Pauly. Framing the issues: Moral distress in health care. *Journal of Health and Human Services Administrations*. 2012. https://link.springer.com/article/10.1007/s10730-012-9176-y.

M. C. Corley. Nurse moral distress: A proposed theory and research agenda. *Nursing Ethics*. 2002; 9(6):636–650.

E. G. Epstein and S. Delgado. Understanding and addressing moral distress. *OJIN: The Online Journal of Issues in Nursing*. 2010; 15(3).

A. Gallagher. Moral distress and moral courage in everyday nursing practice. *OJIN: The Online Journal of Issues in Nursing*. 2010; 16(2).

American Nurses Association. *Code of Ethics for Nurses with Interpretive Statements*. 2015. http://www.nursingworld.org/codeofethics.

Famous holistic doctor & wife allegedly jump to death. 2017. https://www.healthnutnews.com/famous-holistic-doctor-wife-allegedly-jump-to-death.

E. E. Frezza. *Tangled Sutures*. Austin, TX; TMA; 2018. www.texasmedicalassociation.org.

Doctors and stress: The Federation of Medical Societies. http://www.fmshk.org/database/articles/03mb1_3.pdf.

E. E. Frezza. *Medical Ethics*. Routledge; 2018; New York; ISBN # 978-1-138-58107-4.

E. E. Frezza. *The Miserable Doctor*. Ed. Sacramento, CA; Cure Your Practice Press; 2019; ISBN # 978-1-7047-7-3056.

Doctors don't want to be doctors anymore. https://www.apptohealth.com/blog/physician-burnout-career-change/.

Anhedonia. https://www.webmd.com/depression/what-is-anhedonia#1.

"Lack of Professional Appreciation" tops the list of why physicians leave. 2013. http://www.phg.com/2013/04/lack-of-professional-appreciation-tops-the-list-of-why-physicians-leave/.

Chapter 7

Can Malpractice Claims Create Permanent Injury?

In this session we will talk about:

- *Aggressive environment to work in*
- *Distress of lawsuits*
- *Guilty until proven innocent*
- *Communicate with patients*

7.1 Aggressive Environment to Work In

"Why is this happening to physicians? Is that secondary to our increase in chances to bring a lawsuit? I am Jon Perez, an oncology fellow."

Carlo responds. "Unfortunately, most patients do not understand science; they know manners. They look at your office and observe whether it is clean, whether you look professional and have a friendly, adept staff. They ask how long will it take to schedule the next meeting and are concerned if they have to wait too long for appointments, etc. (1).

The doctors who make a positive impression on patients usually are, as you can see in my next slide, those who:

■ Appear unrushed
■ Show interest in the patient as a person
■ Speak in a friendly and not condescending tone

Physicians with these qualities tend to be rarely sued even if they cannot do surgery properly or do not prescribe the correct medicines and clinical pathways.

A dangerous environment exists today in the USA (2, 3). As you can see in my next slide, statistics show the percentages of physicians who have undergone at least one law suit:

■ The first claim by 45 years of age   – 65%
  – Highest risk specialties (surgery, anesthesia, emergency department, obstetrics)   – 88%
  – Lowest risk specialties (family practice, internal medicine)   – 36%

■ The first claim by 65 years old
  – Highest risk specialties   – 99%
  – Lowest risk specialties   – 75%"

7.2 Distress of a Lawsuit

"Wow, that is impressive! I am Dr. Horn from Pathology. But how does the physician react to this?"

"Good question," replies Carlo. "More than 95% of physicians react to being sued by experiencing periods of distress. In my next slide, you can see some of the processes schematically:

■ Most malpractice cases are settled or dismissed
■ About 2% of claims go to court
■ Physicians win about 75% of the time

■ Payments above policy limits rarely, if ever, come from a physician's assets, especially when physicians have policy limits equal to or greater than $500,000"

"I guess that is a lot to take for anyone; I am Dr. Jordan, the dean of the school. How can we see the effects? Are there any side effects?"

"Yes, many," replies Carlo. "As you can see in the next slide, physicians experience a mix of emotions and a range of side effects, most commonly:

■ Anger
■ Frustration
■ Insomnia
■ Denial
■ Guilt/shame
■ Feelings of betrayal
■ Loss of self-esteem
■ Isolation
■ Physical illness
■ Substance abuse
■ Depression/suicide risk
■ Risk of ethical violations"

7.3 Guilty till Proven Innocent

"Physicians facing a malpractice claim will be personally angry; they will become disillusioned and develop a global mistrust of patients. They start to magnify self-doubts and question their competence. They feel depressed and cynical, isolated, frustrated, and unjustly singled out. They start thinking about changing their practice, leaving medicine, and suicide and become intolerant toward patients. Most important, they start changing their attitudes toward their relationships with friends and family.

Most challenging of all is that society considers you guilty until proven innocent! That's what it feels like to be accused of something in this country. No, I didn't go to jail, but if I had indeed been seen as innocent, I wouldn't have lost everything I'd built up either. 'Innocent until proven guilty' is profoundly flawed. For instance, when I was served with a lawsuit, everyone looked at me like I was a criminal. It doesn't matter if the problem was someone else's. It doesn't matter if the accusation was false. It doesn't even matter if the charge wasn't all that damning. Once people start looking at you like you're a pariah, you're a pariah. Sometimes I think I could have committed murder and been treated better."

Out of nowhere everybody started applauding him. That made Carlo feel right about his talk, more in his normal environment; maybe later he could talk about his own experience.

"I am Dr. Richfield from the medicine department. How can we protect ourselves from malpractice claims? Is there any protection?"

Carlo responds, "The straight answer is no. Nobody protects us; we need to protect ourselves by doing better documentation – that is the key. Then we can do the following:

- Implement a strategy in patient regimens.
- Maintain a good relationship with nurses and receptionists.
- Be proactive: send a letter, make phone calls for follow-up, etc."

7.4 Communicate with Patients

"Communicate effectively with your patients. Try to make them understand why they are there, the goals for their care and treatment, and possible outcomes. Treat the patient as a friend, not as a lower class of citizen. Even if you think patients will not understand the science, try to create a scenario that they can understand and that avoids any impression of talking down to them.

- To help ensure proper follow-up, one excellent strategy to implement in your patient regimen is a discussion period with the patient before he or she leaves the office or hospital following surgery.
- It is essential to record a follow-up in writing, sending one copy home with the patient and keeping a second copy in the chart, with documentation that follow-up discussion was given to the patient.
- Doctors also need to encourage patients to make the next appointments before they leave the office. This is easily accomplished if the office is set up with an electronic system; follow-up phone calls are much more difficult in an office that is not computerized.
- Nurses and receptionists are an integral part of your team. As they become more involved in patient care, they play an increasingly vital role in ensuring a comprehensive follow-up.
- The best defense against an attorney who plans to sue you for negligence on follow-up with a patient is to demonstrate that there has been quality communication and proper documentation of the fact that all efforts were made to complete follow-up on the patient.
- Your attorney can thus argue that the patient understood the recommendation but failed to follow the physician's advice.
- Unfortunately, if this is not documented in the progress notes, this argument cannot be made in your defense.
- Many juries assume the physician has superior knowledge and should take steps to ensure the patient is complying, even though this is not a simple task to accomplish.
- While most agree that patients must take responsibility for their healthcare, some juries think that it is solely the doctor who must make sure that the patient complies with follow-up.

◼ They reach this conclusion without taking into consideration how much work this involves, how many patients you have, and how limited your personnel is."

References

1. C. Cecchini. A stigma no physician can afford. *Bag of Pediatrics*; 2018. http://bagofpediatricks.com/2018/02/22/a-stigma-no-physician-can-afford.
2. D. McCullough. You've been served: Lawsuit survival tips for physicians. 2017. https://www.thedoctors.com/articles/youve-been-served-lawsuit-survival-tips-for-physicians/.
3. J. D. Bowen Berry. The physician's guide to medical malpractice. *Proc (Bayl Univ Med Cent)*; 2001; 14(1):109–112. https://www.ncbi.nlm.nih.gov/pmc/articles/PMC1291321/ doi: 10.1080/08998280.2001.11927742.

Suggested Reading

E. E. Frezza. *The Health Care Collapse*. New York; Routledge; 2018; ISBN # 978-1-138-58110-4.

E. L. Vliet. Physician suicide rates have climbed since Obamacare passed. *Physician News Digest*; 2019. https://physiciansnews.com/2015/05/19/physician-suicide-rates-have-climbed-since-obamacare-passed/.

E. E. Frezza. *Tangled Sutures*. Austin, TX; TMA; 2018. www.texasmedicalassociation.org.

J. G. W. S Wong. Doctors and stress. The Federation of Medical Societies. *Medical Bulletin*; 2008; 13(6). http://www.fmshk.org/database/articles/03mb1_3.pdf.

E. E. Frezza. *Medical Ethics*. New York; Routledge; 2018; ISBN # 978-1-138-58107-4.

S. Talbot and W. Dean. Physicians aren't 'burning out.' They're suffering from moral injury. *Stat News*; 2018. https://www.statnews.com/2018/07/26/physicians-not-burning-out-they-are-suffering-moral-injury.

E. E. Frezza. *The Miserable Doctor*. Sacramento, CA; Cure Your Practice Press; 2019; ISBN # 978-1-7047-7-3056.

Chapter 8

Why Is Medicine Burning Out Physicians?

In this session we will talk about:

- *Financial pressures*
- *Hamster in a wheel*
- *Lack of respect toward physicians*

8.1 Financial Pressures

"Mr. Diehl here again. Why is medicine burning out physicians?"

"Well, as you know healthcare is burning out everybody. The average CEO lifespan in a hospital is 2.2 years. So even administrators in healthcare are feeling the problems. Coming back to your question, I can tell you that we are not preparing for this. There is a need for increased discussion and preventive measures for physicians about suicide, a concern that started in medical school and follows the person during the entire professional career.

Why do more physicians see suicide as their only option? The financial pressures play significant roles:

- More patients need to be seen per hour to make ends meet
- Lower payments
- Cumbersome electronic medical systems
- Longer delays in being compensated
- Decreases in patient visits secondary to higher co-pays and deductibles

Financial stress is a known trigger as revenues shrink and overhead costs go up. The higher the administrative and paperwork burden, the more it takes time away from the satisfaction of helping patients. The 'one-size-fits-all' protocols demanded by insurance and government 'guidelines' have been a moral death for most physicians, with subsequent reports and regulations that no one understands, but with substantial financial penalties and even prison if any errors are made. If this is not enough the media report of 'greedy doctors' as indicated by insurance companies, government, and media had been the death penalty for most physicians."

8.2 Hamster in a Wheel

"Doctors are human, too, and have feelings. I think other critically overlooked factors in the rising suicide rates since 2010 include:

- The increasing sense that doctors are just a 'hamster in a wheel,' interchangeable with those having less training and expertise. They are not. I have been fighting for years; everyone in the healthcare system is not equal; in the way chefs make a difference in a restaurant we make a difference in the hospital. The patient follows the doctors, not the hospital.

- Feeling unappreciated by patients, who toss them aside like an old toy when insurance plans change.
- Frustration with patients who dismiss medical recommendations if 'it is not covered by my insurance.'
- Loss of autonomy, control, and independence as faceless insurance clerks, bean-counters, licensing boards, and government agencies dictate how, where, and when the medicine is to be practiced, with no knowledge of the patient in question."

8.3 Lack of Respect toward Physicians

"After years of hard work, helping countless thousands of patients and paying taxes through the nose, my reward for being a good citizen and a good human being is to have some greedy lawyer come out from under his rock and start filing unjustifiable lawsuits against me. He thought he would build a name for himself; he failed. He told his client he would make them rich. He had to face them when that didn't happen.

Where is the respect? Where is basic human dignity? Where is the integrity? He filed a poorly informed lawsuit in a half-baked attempt to make a lot of money, and he rightly failed. The medical equivalent would be the surgeon who removes healthy organs just to get paid for doing the surgery. It is barbaric, disrespectful, and dangerous. Did he check the case? Did he check out the other surgeon's job? Did he have another opinion on him and me? Did they review the literature? So many unanswered questions.

Metrics, measurement systems, to partially determine the quality of care are a good idea. If they were set up by people who know how the medical system works, they could accomplish a lot. Currently, an elective cholecystectomy can be evaluated against emergency pancreatitis treatment. They are not the same. There are metrics for doctors but not for lawyers, for example. While the surgical procedures may be the same, no two patients are alike, and that is why this metric evaluation concept has limited potential; and each case needs to be evaluated independently.

I attended court a few times to see how these lawsuits are handled, and sometimes the attorneys will say the most uninformed things to win a case. First of all, their client is never at fault, period. Apparently, in the magical land of the tort lawyer, only one party is ever at fault for any problem, and that party is never their party. I heard one attorney say 'Oh but a physician is more intelligent. Therefore it is his fault because he is supposed to tell the patient what to do and how to do it.' I am better educated than almost all of my patients on the issue they came to me for. That's how that works. That's why we go to professionals. As to intelligence, the only intelligence one can surmise about here is the lawyer's, and he doesn't come out looking too swift after saying things like that. This lawyer also seemed to forget that my intelligence and my training combined cannot be responsible for the patient's decisions, actions, or responses to my words."

"It is a society that blames each other," commented Jeremy.

"Yes, you are right," continued Carlo. "You don't get to blame me for your lack of discipline because I am educated differently than you. You don't get to blame me for your lack of self-care because you perceive me as smarter than you. Your choices are never someone else's fault, never, and suing someone else because of your bad decisions is bad for you, bad for them, and bad for our society.

Healthcare is not a casino. It is not Las Vegas. It's not even church bingo. You don't get to try your luck suing professionals until you get lucky and can retire on your winnings. Some lawyers try to make the tort system look like some casino. Those who do are two-armed bandits using you to line their wallets. After expenses and taxes, almost all lawsuit recipients receive very little for their trouble.

It's hard to build a good life while remaining the victim all the time. Notice that, outside of the movies, very few people make a comfortable living off of lawsuits.

Yes, there is a place in society for lawsuits, but this undignified, self-destructive pattern of living off of them is not it. When a professional does their best, informs you, and gives you the benefit of their education and training toward your well-being, have the dignity to provide them with the chance to make any problem right before considering a lawsuit.

I don't believe that there are malicious physicians out there, I don't think physicians try purposely to hurt patients, but I do believe that there are a lot of patients who try deliberately to hurt the physician because that is the only income that they have. That is why I have been working mostly in Texas, where the laws protect the physician somewhat more than in other states.

In certain US states, our freedom extends to the freedom to have discussions about the end of life. There are states you can go to and apply for assisted suicide. It is your decision; it is your respected decision in this free society. Some states support assisted suicide; some states don't. Some states support abortion; some states don't. The freedoms of this country are remarkable. Even when one state won't do as you want, another will. Where else can you find that in one nation?

There is so much freedom in the United States, and the people who are born and raised here don't understand what they have. They don't understand God's gift that they have because they were born in America.

I was not born in America. I decided to come to America as an adult. I know what freedom means. People who were born in America have no clue about what a big gift they received by being born here."

Suggested Reading

Patients mistreating doctors. *Medical Summary*, Volume 39. 1917. https://books.google.com/books?id=7B4CAAAAYAAJ&pg =PA51&lpg=PA51&dq=do+doctor+feels+like+chicken +in+a+wheel&source=bl&ots=4a4ANQ3Ogo&amp ;sig=ACfU3U2R6lZ_2A2Y4wKcj3CQa7ObS5RgpA&hl=en& amp;sa=X&ved=2ahUKEwjojNuv0oPnAhXUuZ4KHQ8 MBNIQ6AEwCXoECAgQAQ#v=onepage&q=do%20doctor %20feels%20like%20chicken%20in%20a%20wheel&f=false.

Amy Paturel. When the perpetrators are patients. Special to AAMCNews, October 23, 2018. https://www.aamc.org/news-insi ghts/when-perpetrators-are-patients.

Ahmad Yousaf. With doctors losing respect, perhaps it's time to expose medicine's dark side. May 22, 2016. https://www.kev inmd.com/blog/2016/05/with-doctors-losing-respect-perhaps-its -time-to-expose-medicines-dark-side.html.

E. E. Frezza. *The Health Care Collapse*. New York; Routledge; 2018; ISBN # 978-1-138-58110-4.

E. L. Vliet. Physician suicide rates have climbed since Obamacare passed. *Physician News Digest*; 2019. https://physiciansnews.co m/2015/05/19/physician-suicide-rates-have-climbed-since-obam acare-passed/.

E. E. Frezza. *Tangled Sutures*. Austin, TX; TMA; 2018. www.texasme dicalassociation.org.

J. G. W. S. Wong. Doctors and stress. The Federation of Medical Societies. *Medical Bulletin*; 2008; 13(6). http://www.fmshk.org/ database/articles/03mb1_3.pdf.

E. E. Frezza. *Medical Ethics*. New York; Routledge; 2018; ISBN # 978-1-138-58107-4.

S. Talbot and W. Dean. Physicians aren't 'burning out.' They're suffering from moral injury. *Stat News*; 2018. https://www.statnews .com/2018/07/26/physicians-not-burning-out-they-are-suffering -moral-injury.

E. E. Frezza. *The Miserable Doctor*. Sacramento, CA; Cure Your Practice Press; 2019; ISBN # 978-1-7047-7-3056.

Chapter 9

Broken Systems and Culture

In this session we will talk about:

- *Corporate culture*
- *Increasing denial of insurance services*
- *Refusing clinical evidence*
- *Locum company cartels*

9.1 Corporate Culture

"What are the most difficult things for you to deal with? Can you lose your mind like in the movie *The Shining* with Jack Nicholson? I am Bob, chief resident in medicine."

"It is a funny question Bob, but a good one. If I have to think about something, I will say corporate culture. Many corporations are buying more and more hospitals, which is resulting in rules and restrictions on everyone, including physicians.

Corporate culture is a beast unto itself. Something the hospital corporations will do is ask if you've had any lawsuits in the past five years. I said no, none in five years. Then they came back later and said that I didn't tell them about the lawsuit from 20 years ago. That lawsuit was 20 years ago, not five. So now I report every single lawsuit at the beginning, so they can't do that again.

Sometimes when you need help to fill out an application, you find people who have no idea how to help you. They don't have any clue. This happens in hospitals and offices all the time. You are directed to people who are lower and lower on the hierarchy until your request doesn't even make sense to the person you ask. They won't admit that, so they'll say they can't help you and then stonewall you.

Health insurance companies have mastered this. You always get a secretary or operator. These people are what they are because often they cannot do better. Whatever you do, don't try to make a conversation when you're asking for help. Government being what it is, it's not unusual to find people in higher positions without a clue either.

The medical literature abounds with a variety of controversial issues that are intertwined between the physician and the healthcare system. It would be impossible to adequately reveal or address all of these issues in a single conference. In the following, I would like to list some of the more current and controversial issues that challenge physicians in their relationship with the ever-changing healthcare system.

As the health insurance industry has increased in size and power, it has been able to impact medical care by the ability to pay for or deny benefits for specific procedures and conditions. Inherent in the creation of some healthcare products, such as HMOs or PPOs, is the need for cost containment and efficiency. In applying this to the sheltered lives that they insure, healthcare insurers have not paid for some services and procedures that the physician may deem necessary for the treatment or prevention of a medical condition. Most notably has been the persistent denial of preventive medicine and screening tests by some insurers, which ultimately may be more cost-effective but do not bring any short-term reductions in expenses. By their private ownership, many healthcare insurers have the same constraints of profitability and growth that other private industries do. This sometimes forces the healthcare insurance industry to choose between what expenses they can cover, which in the case of preventive medicine often is removed from the budget."

9.2 Increasing Denial of Insurance Services

"In some cases (i.e., colonoscopy after a right colon cancer was missed in President Ronald Regan by doing only a sigmoidos-copy), it has required legislation to force the health insurance industry to provide necessary screening and prevention pro-cedures. Physicians can be put in an awkward position if they recommend a procedure or treatment that they feel is essen-tial for the appropriate care of the patient when the patient's insurer will not cover that expense. Also, physicians who work for organizations that provide health insurance products may repeatedly be informed of the need for cost containment and the payment of therapy. They can be discouraged from making appropriate out-of-network referrals or prescribing necessary treatments due to the lack of cost containment.

In some cases, physicians derive direct personal benefits (i.e., salary bonuses), which are based on the profitability of the providing organization. The inherent conflicts in this situa-tion are apparent. In some cases, circumstances regarding cov-erage of benefits have required litigation to achieve resolution.

I had a manager from a former practice who was not very well oriented to his office job. I had to go to him for all the reimbursement and all the questions in the office. I dared not go to the hospital, nor to the other administrator. So when I started, the office was not set up yet. I waited for two months, and in the end, I moved the furniture myself and fixed the room so I could see patients. I waited for three months to have a key to the office, and I had been waiting for more than four months to get reimbursement. Organizational policy stated that I must go through him to be reimbursed.

He didn't respond to emails. He didn't respond to regular mail. He didn't respond to texts. He didn't respond to phone calls, and when I tried to talk to him, he said 'yes, yes, yes,' but nothing ever happened. I spoke to the administration. I spoke to higher-ups, and nothing happened. He is a soft-spoken man. He is nice. He never challenged the system, and so the system has let him get away with doing nothing. Because he is a nice guy, I have to work in an unfurnished office? No bed, no blood pressure machine to check patients. On top of this, they were complaining because patients were not coming!"

9.3 Refusing Clinical Evidence

"I had a pediatric patient who came in 10 days after a dog bite, and unfortunately, his wound became infected. I had to do something about it. I learned that I could not use lidocaine in my office to numb the area. Since I am a surgeon, I use a lot of lidocaine. The only person in the office who could use lidocaine, according to the manager of the clinic, was the nurse practitioner.

The nurse practitioner is, according to him, a wound specialist. He's never treated a wound, never sutured, never actually opened and closed any skin, but he is a wound specialist. Meanwhile I, the surgeon, am not the wound specialist and I am not allowed to use lidocaine. This insanity has been following me all this time where I work in hospitals and clinics.

How can you expect a person to do their job if you have people like this? Heaven forbid I should tell them how I feel about the situation. Thinking myself qualified to do wound care made me an instant pariah. This has got to be the lowest level of inner-office politics I have ever run across.

You cannot be kind enough for these people. They lack fundamental respect or understanding of who is paying the bills and why they are working in the office. They don't work in the office because it is under their name.

God save anybody if we make any comments because then it's taken as derogatory. It is going to be sexual harassment, even if it is nothing sexual. There is always going to be an excuse for their mediocrity.

That manager? He's still there. He has been moved from managing the clinic to controlling the flow of the patients in the hospital. He hired a manager for the office. The manager he hired is just like him. This manager has no clue how to manage anything. So again, if in this case, someone says something, they get reported. Why do physicians put themselves in this condition? Why do we have to go through life with this stress of other people telling us what to do? When they have no clue how to run a clinic or a floor patient. I think that society has been losing its point.

Everybody seems to think they deserve everything. They don't go to school. They don't get an education. They seem to think working in the same office with highly trained professionals gives them equal professional status. Everybody should be respected as an equal. But when skill levels are different, each skillset should be recognized for its own merits. If they can't do that, then they are probably in the wrong job.

Most care facilities and most hospitals are owned by corporations. Corporations provide certain insulation of liability that allows the officers to rest comfortably in their policy setting and their responses to legal challenges. For a lawyer suing, a corporation is a greater challenge. The professionals, the highly paid individuals, are the low-hanging fruit for tort attorneys.

When the attorneys know everyone in town, we professionals who are new to the area have no rights. Sure we have legal rights, but enforcing them is nearly impossible. When you are responsible for the office, but you have no right to take a stand or to establish a policy or to respond to potential threats, it is impossible to remain active for long."

9.4 Locum Company Cartels

"Hello, I am Riccardo. I am a fellow in Laparoscopy, and I am trying to find a shift and night job to supplement my fellow salary since I have two children. What about just working for locum companies, so you don't have to deal with all of that?"

"I wish I had something positive to say," replied Carlo, "I have lived in fear of having to work for a locum tenens company to remain employed. It is a black hole of career oblivion for those who succumb. Included in their contract is the stipulation that their clients and the hospitals they work with can never develop a permanent relationship. Many temporary employment agencies in the broader business world work to get their clients into long-term positions and consider such relationships proof of their success and business skills.

Do you know that if you were presented by a locum company to a hospital that the locum company can keep tabs on you for two years, yes two, not just the hospital but the entire corporation system? You are stuck as a prisoner, and you do not even know!!

Locum tenens companies are only there for the dollar and for the corporations. They minimize the risk of lawsuits, not by providing excellent care and professionalism, or by long-term relationship building, but by obfuscation and confusion in paperwork. Their lawyers could lose a cruise ship in a bathtub!

It is right to protect your business's ability to continue to serve in the best way possible. It is unethical and wrong to defend your business's ability to keep making money at all costs. We work in a profession of life and death. Quality of care must come first.

I would advise people just entering a profession to prepare for such eventualities. You never know when an outside influence could come crashing down on your head, ruining the plans you had so carefully wrought. Be prepared for the time when you lose all negotiating power, perhaps with an alternative career that will allow you to continue earning well, probably in politics if you don't mind getting your hands irreversibly dirty. You can lose your leverage at any moment. Think ahead like I didn't."

Suggested Reading

Barbara Gardner Cook. Redefining corporate medicine. *Family Practice Management.* 1999; 6(9):9. https://www.aafp.org/fpm/1999/1000/p9.html.

What is a clinical manager? https://www.jobhero.com/what-is-a-clinic-manager/.

Medical office manager: Job description. https://www.verywellhealth.com/medical-office-manager-job-description-2317265.

Melissa DeCapua. The importance of Locum Tenens in modern healthcare. 2017. https://www.healthecareers.com/article/career/locum-tenens-modern-healthcare.

E. E. Frezza. *The Health Care Collapse.* New York; Routledge; 2018; ISBN # 978-1-138-58110-4.

E. L. Vliet. Physician suicide rates have climbed since Obamacare passed. *Physician News Digest;* 2015. https://physiciansnews.com/2015/05/19/physician-suicide-rates-have-climbed-since-obamacare-passed/.

E. E. Frezza. *Tangled Sutures.* TMA; 2018. www.texasmedicalassociation.org.

J. G. W. S. Wong. Doctors and stress. The Federation of Medical Societies. *Medical Bulletin;* 2018. http://www.fmshk.org/database/articles/03mb1_3.pdf.

E. E. Frezza. *Medical Ethics.* New York; Routledge; 2018; ISBN # 978-1-138-58107-4.

S. Talbot and W. Dean. Physicians aren't 'burning out.' They're suffering from moral injury. 2018. https://www.statnews.com/2018/07/26/physicians-not-burning-out-they-are-suffering-moral-injury.

E. E. Frezza. *The Miserable Doctor.* Sacramento, CA; Cure Your Practice Press; 2019; ISBN # 978-1-7047-7-3056.

Chapter 10

Physicians Leaving Medicine

In this session we will talk about:

- *Lost goals*
- *Medicine is an art, not just a business*

10.1 Lost Goals

"Here I am again, the dean. What do you mean looking for another career, leaving medicine after all the sacrifice? I don't want you to share with my medical students."

Carlo smiles and presents a few slides. "Physicians like to become entrepreneurs since they experience:

1. Lost goals
2. Lost control of the healthcare
3. Loss of recognition from healthcare administration

Christina Farr made an excellent point on physicians changing jobs:

> It's a challenge to quantify the exact number of doctors moving out of healthcare into the tech world. Even if a large physicians' group like the American Medical Association (AMA) tried to keep track, it would need to determine whether to include doctors that advise startups but still practice one or two days a week or just those who have left medicine altogether. I suspect that the former category is much more extensive. Suffice it to say, though, that Weiss is far from alone–the migration of doctors into the health tech space is noticeable. (1)
>
> It is now fairly common for well-funded health-tech startups to have medical directors, physician founders, or chief medical/health officers on their team. Some high-profile examples include Collective Health, Sherpaa, Startup Health, Doximity, Aledade, and AthenaHealth. And the AMA tells me it is pro-actively forging partnerships in Silicon Valley and beyond to help doctors "work in tandem on the innovative tech solutions that promise to change health care. (2)

Web-based companies, manufacturers, and pharmaceutical, and other companies have catered to doctors with experience in high tech and brought the problems to the surface (3).

A few California-based doctors started a private Facebook group called 'dropout docs.' This includes: Rebecca Coelius, a UCSF medical school graduate who worked as a health director at Code for America; Amanda Angelotti, a fellow UCSF graduate who works in clinical systems design at One Medical; Sean Duffy, a Harvard Medical School dropout who cofounded Omada Health; and Connie Chen, a practicing doctor who cofounded a chronic disease management app called Vida. This is bringing the problems the doctors have today: to be or not to be a doctor? This is the question many asked today, after many years of training and extensive payments of medical school loans (4, 5)."

10.2 Medicine Is an Art, Not Just a Business

"The present state of the healthcare profession has been increasing the push to get out of medicine. Some of the problems are:

1. Depression
2. Loss of patient recognition since the public believes that taking care of them is a 'must' we need to do with or without being paid for it
3. Practicing medicine in the role of a secretary and the loss of the art of our profession

All of these issues and more have brought burnout to physicians and their suicide rate is higher than ever; doctors are getting tired, and they want to do something else."

"Hello, here I am again, the chair of medicine. Why do you think this is happening so often? What was the initial trigger?"

Carlo answered: "Doctors hate insurance companies because they often feel they are powerless when it comes to dealing with them. The average physician insurance contract is written entirely in favor of the insurance company. The insurance company gets to decide what is medically necessary, how disputes are resolved, and how much the physician is to be paid. When it comes to payment, the physician usually, unless he or she is with a large group, has very little negotiating power. Often the insurance company unilaterally changes significant contract terms with a single written notice to the physician that requires no independent physician agreement.

Insurance companies also affiliate or purchase other contracts. When this happens, a physician will suddenly be subject to a reduction in rates with a company he previously had no agreement with because he has a deal with another. There is nothing the physician can do in response to this except to seek to terminate the agreement, which is extremely difficult to do. Did I answer your point?"

"Yes," said the chair of medicine.

References

1. N. Spector. The doctor is out? Why physicians are leaving their practices to pursue other careers. *NBC News*; 2019. https://www.nbcnews.com/business/business-news/doctor-out-why-physicians-are-leaving-their-practices-pursue-other-n900921.
2. Why so many doctors are advising startups. *Fast Company*. https://www.fastcompany.com/3059231/why-so-many-doctors-are-advising-startups.
3. Drop out doc. Thousands of doctors want to join. https://money.cnn.com/2015/10/30/smallbusiness/dropout-club-for-doctors/index.html; Instagram page. https://www.instagram.com/dropoutdoc/?hl=en.
4. The drop out doctor community. https://www.statnews.com/2017/05/24/doctors-burnout-online-community/.
5. Drop out and counseling. https://www.scientificamerican.com/article/in-drop-out-club-doctors-counsel-one-another-on-quitting-the-field/.

Chapter 11

Impossible Victory: Physicians Are the New Chain Worker

In this session we will talk about:

- *Managers who lack clinical training*
- *Managers and physicians with opposing aims*
- *How medicine is not a cookbook*

11.1 Managers Who Lack Clinical Training

"But why have we arrived at this point, Dr. Bruni? Here, on the back left, I am Charles Koss, cardiothoracic surgeon fellow."

Carlo then answered, "What do you call it when a practice offers a new doctor a good salary but provides no patients, no marketing, and no clinic setup? What do you call it when the practice has few operating rooms and a two-bed intensive care unit, and the staff are not trained on how to handle patients? As the doctor in question, I call it an impossible victory and a sign of disaster.

What do you do, as a surgeon, when a board member of the practice tells you that you are supposed to sit in your office and be available for walk-in patients? I explained that they are confusing the job of a family doctor with the job of a surgeon. I showed them that I have been on call every day since I started work for them. I showed them that my name and contact information are in the emergency room, as well. I am literally on call twenty-four hours a day, seven days a week, and that is why my job is not structured like a family doctor.

I was sitting with three board members, two men and a woman, and we were discussing my performance. They said that I didn't sit in my office enough. I told them about the difference between a family physician and a surgeon and asked them, 'Why do I want to sit in my office when I don't have an office? I have a closet that was assigned as an office, no window, just room enough to walk in and out and not even room to put another chair. What am I going to do in the office as a surgeon?' People don't stop into a surgeon's office and say 'Hey, by the way, I need my gallbladder out.'

Did they understand? I genuinely don't think they had any desire to understand. They never responded.

The next thing they said, something such people usually say, was, 'You are too focused on doing medical administration.'

I said nothing, but I thought, 'do you know that your office manager doesn't know the difference between a clinic run by a family physician, an internist, a gastroenterologist, or a surgeon?'

They looked like deer in the headlights. When I realized that I was getting nowhere with them, I just said, 'I think you need a medical officer to explain to your staff and others how to run a hospital, to explain to you the difference between surgery, medicine, and family practice.'

What do you call it when the practice is run by a rarely present physician who talks the talk but doesn't walk the walk? When he makes big promises and never delivers, what do you call that? When you try to hold him to his promise, and his only response is, 'We can't work together'? This is an impossible victory."

11.2 Managers and Physicians Have Opposing Aims

"Why should a physician ever need to hear the explanation that a surgeon makes money for the hospital in the operating room? Why would a physician ever think that a surgeon's time is better spent doing administrative work? It's simple business math. Anybody can write policies. Indeed, the surgeon and all other practitioners should review the plans and give feedback so that effective policies can be adopted, but the surgeon doesn't bring income to the practice behind a desk. That is why hospitals fight to name surgeons chief medical officer unless they are retired.

What do you call it when a nurse is a CEO and then suddenly becomes the chief operations officer of the practice? That is not a promotion. That is an impossible victory. And this, unfortunately, is the common ground where physicians have to work every day. The CEO, she messed up the SWOT (strengths, weaknesses, opportunities, and threats) analysis as to why they needed a surgeon and identifying the referral base of patients they can offer to sustain the surgeon's salary. If it were in a different business, she would be fired right there. Unfortunately, she saved herself changing jobs, and the surgeon lost the job!

We physicians were solely responsible for the mess created by inept administration people that are so afraid of confrontation that they instead prefer to have an excellent 'yes man' than an excellent physician. In healthcare, you cannot be a yes man since your decisions affect other human beings.

So, I don't have enough RVUs (relative value units) because I don't have patients coming to the clinic. Might that have to do with the fact that there are not enough family physicians in town to refer patients? Might it have to do with the fact that there aren't enough nurse practitioners in town to refer patients?

How can it be possible that a specialty clinic can see more patients than a family practice clinic in a town that has a shortage of family physicians? How is it possible that you can set up a practice when nobody knows that you are in town? How is it possible that the marketing is done with the name of the company, but not with the doctor's name, so nobody knows who the doctor is? How is it that your first marketing effort started three months after the clinic opened? How is it that the doctor doesn't even get a key to his own office until two months after he's hired? And the big question: how can they honestly expect to make any money from a clinic that was that poorly organized from the start?

Rural health is the answer! Even if there is not much work, the corporation gets paid by patient headcount, not by the severity of the disease. The hospital can charge this way, but a private physician practice cannot!"

11.3 Medicine Is Not a Cook Book

"The question marks have been replaced with exclamation marks! A good victory for the hospital but an impossible victory for a physician.

My advice to all physicians is if you see any signs of inconsistency, self-destructive policies, or board members that haven't a clue, run away before the corporation of the day decides that you are not a valuable physician because you don't make enough money for the hospital.

The real questions are who did this SWOT analysis before hiring me?

Who assured the board, the corporation, and the hospital board that hiring a physician would be a favorable, remunerative deal and that you would have enough patients to support the practice?

Those people that did the SWOT analysis, those people that approved the physician position, those are the ones that need to be fired. Maybe the SWOT analysis was based on the assumption that the board would have an organized and accountable team setting up the clinic, though. Still, if ever you are offered a job by a barrel full of monkeys masquerading as a hospital board, run! Run away!"

The audience applauded again in a sign of support and agreement. Even the administrators agreed that it was weird.

"This is impossible," said Dr. Smooth, the vice dean for medical affairs.

"How can it be?" Carlo answered. "Working at the university is different from a small hospital? Maybe not. Lack of personnel, people who want to go home, a union that gives them the right of being lazy, instead of checking if they do their work. Unions will be stronger if they defend the people who work and help the lazy ones to get up, otherwise they will never have strength and no one will use union personnel. Businesspeople in charge of the clinic business who are not prepared follow clinical rules, just as an apprentice chef follows recipes in a 'cookbook' while not understanding the location and business, and they don't want to admit to how they know, even if they don't."

Suggested Reading

J. Doroshow. Cookbook medicine is a recipe for disaster. *Huffpost*, 2013. https://www.huffpost.com/entry/cookbook-medicine_b _2792900.

Stanford Medical School. Every patient is different. Different reporting of the same issues. 2019. https://stanfordhealthcare.org/abou t-us/quality.html.

Arthur H. Gale. The hospital as a factory and the physician as an assembly line worker. *Missouri Medicine*. 2016; 113(1):7–9. https ://www.ncbi.nlm.nih.gov/pmc/articles/PMC6139751/.

E. E. Frezza. *The Health Care Collapse*. New York; Routledge; 2018; ISBN # 978-1-138-58110-4.

E. E. Frezza. *Tangled Sutures*. Austin, TX; TMA; 2018. www.texasme dicalassociation.org.

E. E. Frezza. *Medical Ethics*. New York, Routledge; 2018; ISBN # 978-1-138-58107-4.

E. E. Frezza. *The Miserable Doctor*. Sacramento, CA; Cure Your Practice Press; 2019; ISBN # 978-1-7047-7-3056.

Chapter 12

Emotional Trauma: Brain Zapping and Concussion

In this session we will talk about:

- *Emotional trauma*
- *The similar symptoms of concussion and moral distress*
- *Brain zapping*

12.1 Emotional Trauma

"Do you think we should include emotional trauma as a cause of moral injury? Is there a physical effect? I am Dr. Liam. I am a family physician, and these emotional injuries should be included in workman's compensation issues as a work-related disease.

Is it something I need to be aware of one day since I see a lot of workman's compensation injuries? It seems, from the beginning of your talk, that moral distress syndrome includes a wide variety of physical and mental diseases, but does it include emotional injuries?"

"Yes, there are too many symptoms and too many side effects that the medical societies and the insurance companies should soon include as workman's comp since they are work-related injuries. Anecdotally, there is something else I would like to tell you, which was my direct experience," responded Carlo, "but it is anecdotal and is not scientific proof yet.

First, I was diagnosed with angina and suffered a mild case of angina pectoris, and my blood pressure was also out of control. Now I am on medication. I can't even imagine what the side effects on my brain are. I felt I suffered from a brain injury, as well."

12.2 The Similar Symptoms of Concussion and Moral Distress

"Maybe an autopsy should be done on people with moral distress. Perhaps we will discover another disease. This definitely will create lots of lawsuits. I am talking about emotional concussion. I think emotional commotion has similarities to what was found in football players, micro-concussion, which eventually replaces the brain cell with amyloid material. Would any researchers in advance be interested in performing my autopsy?" The crowd laughs.

"I am glad that you are alive, I guess," said Diana Perez from Pediatrics.

"Thanks Diana. I don't think it's an issue at this point. I've died several times in my heart, in my mind, but I never put a gun to my head like my poor boss.

What is sad about my old boss is that 'the dark forces' of the organization made his family guilty; they killed him. The dark side took over! He was accused of fraud, of hiring substandard physicians, of stealing money from the Veteran Hospital, by the university, and he could not take it and shot himself. Many times, the dark side has knocked on my door, but I survived my lost tangled life!

It is difficult for the human mind to escape the past. Thinking about escaping the past brings it into sharp focus. It's like being a football player who gets hit several times and develops a degenerative disease that makes you crazy. It's the emotional traumas that are like concussions. While watching the Will Smith football movie *Concussion*, it occurred to me that there are some similarities between life stresses and being physically tackled on the football field.

Emotional trauma makes a mark, a scar in your brain, which will never heal. Injuries don't allow for new tissue to replace the old and result in less brain function. You will lose your balance. You will lose your affect. You become flat not because of emotional detachment but because you can no longer process certain emotions. You become demented. Your synapses are gone, and you are very much gone too. With all the scar tissue and the ensuing damage, you don't care, and your life becomes flat and emotionless. After a while, you look in the mirror and don't recognize the person you see. It's as if there are two people in the mirror. This harms your family too. I find this is equally true for the body. That's why Eastern culture believes in the mind-body balance called 'zen,' and they are healthier for it."

12.3 Brain Zapping

"I still remember distinctly the night that I felt a stabbing in my heart. At the same time, electric shivering passed through my brain while I was thinking about my problems; it also happened while I was at work. My staff was waiting for me.

There's a phenomenon that I've recently learned about called brain zapping. For the first time in my life, I have started feeling small 'lightning strikes' inside my head. I would feel electrical shocks going from one ear to the other, or from my eyes to the bottom of my neck. At first, I would wake up scared and astonished since I didn't know what to make of them. I thought my brain was exploding, or I was about to die. It seems that my brain was overheating.

My wife was asleep next to me, and I didn't want to give her more stress, so I lay there contemplating the ceiling. I took comfort watching the leaves on the trees outside, understanding that life and death are cyclical as trees and their leaves remind us. I was still scared as I had never heard of brain regeneration. I feared I might go into a coma and never wake up. That thought made me keep myself awake, so I wouldn't fall asleep and experience more zapping.

I learned that brain zapping frequently happens to people under very intense stress, and it is not very dangerous. I have more research to do to verify this, but it offers some comfort for now. I still wonder if it might cause the same symptomatology that concussions produce in football players.

These zaps feel as if your head, brain, or both have experienced a sudden shock. It might also feel like a jolt, a tremor, a vibration, or a sudden shake. People frequently describe the experience as feeling like an electric shock jolted them.

Symptoms seem to come out of nowhere and have no medical explanation as yet. They generally last a few seconds when the person is relaxing or is asleep. They can affect a small part of the head or the brain, but they can also affect an entire region. Symptoms can occur anywhere from rarely up to persistently. Zaps can feel just strong enough to notice, all the way up to severe and even painful. Often they seem more prevalent when anxiety or stress is high but have been documented when there were no unusual stressors in the person's life.

Apprehensive behavior creates a state of anxiety. This activates the body's emergency response, the stress response. The stress response secretes stress hormones into the bloodstream where they bring about specific changes. These changes are emotional, psychological, and physiological and help the body to deal with danger. They trigger the fight, flight, or freeze response. The stress response is often called the fight or flight response. These biochemical changes can create brain zapping.

As body stressors increase overall, symptoms will get worse. Those symptoms can vary widely by type, number, intensity, duration, and frequency. Brain and head zaps are a typical indication of a persistently elevated stress response. I wonder if, in those people who have had brain zaps but claim no abnormal stressors in their life, higher levels of stress hormones might still be found in blood tests. This can be the next frontier to study in the area of moral distress.

Angina is a more common side effect of stress because you can measure it. I ignored it for a year and finally was diagnosed with angina.

Those same 'dark forces' have approached me many times. I sent them back. I will survive."

Suggested Reading

C. Sippin. Emotional concussion can cause as much damage as physical concussions. 2013. https://acestoohigh.com/2013/06/25/emotional-concussions-can-cause-as-much-damage-as-physical-concussions/.

C. O'Keefe Osborn. The secret of brain shake-brain zapping. 2018. https://www.healthline.com/health/brain-shakes.

Michelle Overman. What causes brain zapping? *Mental Health*; 2019. https://www.e-counseling.com/mental-health/what-are-brain-zaps-and-what-causes-them/.

Mayo Clinic. Angina is stress related. *Mayo Clinic*; 2019. https://www.mayoclinic.org/diseases-conditions/angina/symptoms-causes/syc-20369373.

S. Boyles. Family related stress can cause angina. 2010. https://www.webmd.com/heart-disease/news/20101223/family-stress-linked-to-angina-pain#1.

N. Fitzgerald. How job stress affects your heart. 2019. https://www.webmd.com/heart/features/job-stress-and-your-heart#1.

M. Hitti. Job stress take a toll on your heart. 2019. https://www.webmd.com/heart-disease/news/20080124/job-stress-takes-toll-on-the-heart.

Physical signs of stress. 2019. https://www.webmd.com/balance/stres
s-management/stress-symptoms-effects_of-stress-on-the-body#1.

E. E. Frezza. *The Health Care Collapse*. New York; Routledge; 2018; ISBN # 978-1-138-58110-4.

E. E. Frezza. *Tangled Sutures*. Austin, TX; TMA; 2018. www.texasme dicalassociation.org.

E. E. Frezza. *Medical Ethics*. New York; Routledge; 2018; ISBN # 978-1-138-58107-4.

E. E. Frezza. *The Miserable Doctor*. Sacramento, CA; Cure Your Practice Press; 2019; ISBN # 978-1-7047-7-3056.

Chapter 13

Divorce among Physicians

In this session we will talk about:

- *Physician divorce studies*
- *Specialty traits*
- *Divorce in the USA*
- *Average first marriage duration*
- *Cost for taxpayers*

13.1 Physician Divorce Study

"You mentioned other personal loss; to what other loss are you referring?" asked Dr. Metha.

"Divorce, breaking families, children growing up with a broken family," answered Carlo.

"Do you have any data?" Dr. Metha rebutted.

"Of course," smiled Carlo. "Let me go to the next session of slides from the article by Dr. Anupam Jena and Dr. Dan Ly (1). They analyzed the results of surveys of more than 40,000 doctors and 200,000 nurses, pharmacists, dentists, and health-care executives, conducted between 2008 and 2013.

Those who said they'd been divorced included 23 percent of pharmacists, 24 percent of doctors, 25 percent of dentists, 31 percent of healthcare executives, and 33 percent of nurses.

The researchers also looked at people who work outside the health field and found that 35 percent of them had been divorced (1).

Among doctors, women were about 1.5 times more likely to have been divorced than men of a similar age. Female doctors who worked more than 40 hours a week were more likely to be divorced than those who worked fewer hours, while the reverse was true among male doctors.

The study's lead author, Dr. Dan Ly, explained in the news release, 'We believe that the higher incidence of divorce among female physicians stems from the greater tradeoffs they are forced to make to achieve work/life balance' (2).

'More research is needed to understand whether that interpretation is indeed accurate and, if it is, what can be done to help with work/life balance,' he added (1)."

13.2 Specialty Traits

"Excuse me," said Dr. Haney, "I am a pediatrician, and I thought we were the best match for marriage, but someone told me the opposite. Do you have any data? Is there a direct correlation between divorce and specialties?"

"Unfortunately, yes," replied Carlo. "Physician divorce rates vary by specialty and psychological traits (2). According to the University of Pittsburgh web page:

1. Divorce rates among physicians are not affected by a host of other factors, including gender, which previously was thought to be relevant, according to a study by a University of Pittsburgh assistant professor, Bruce L.

Rollman, published in a March issue of the *New England Journal of Medicine* (3).

2. The overall cumulative rate of divorce among 1,118 physicians was 29 percent over 30 years of marriage. Rollman found that psychiatrists had the highest divorce rate, 50 percent, followed by surgeons, 33 percent. For internists, pediatricians, and pathologists, the rates ranged from 22 to 24 percent.

3. Some psychological variables also proved crucial. Physicians who scored in the highest quarter on a test measuring anger had a 44 percent incidence of divorce compared with 27 percent for the rest of the study group. Perceiving one's self as having been less emotionally close with one's parents was also associated with a higher divorce rate.

4. Rollman's study debunked other factors previously thought to affect divorce among physicians, including gender, depression, religion, medical school class rank, being an only child, parental history of divorce, and having a parent or parents who were physicians. While women physicians had a higher absolute incidence of divorce (37 percent women versus 28 percent men), after adjusting for other factors, such as specialty, female physicians had the same risk of divorce as male physicians (2).

Pediatricians try to be warm and friendly, but at the same time, they mix family issues with their overwhelmed caring feeling for their patients.

When asked to guess which specialty had the highest divorce rate, most physicians said surgeons, who had the second-highest rate.

'Surgeons are never home,' reported Dr. Nada Stotland in 'Medical Specialty and the Incidence of Divorce' published in today's issue of the *New England Journal of Medicine* (March 13, 1997). 'They're abused in their training; it's extremely hierarchical, they're used to giving orders and having them obeyed unquestioningly. Not all spouses are into being surgical nurses' (3).

Rollman Drew was on the Johns Hopkins Precursors Study, which tracked 1,337 people who entered the Johns Hopkins University School from 1944 through 1960. That group included only eight percent female physicians, two percent Asians, and no African-Americans. Excluding those who did not graduate, as well as those for whom marital and divorce information was incomplete, Rollman's study was based on 1,118 married physicians and reported in the *New England Journal of Medicine* (4)."

13.3 Divorce in the USA

"It is astonishing," commented Dr. Haney, "I am Joyce, a medical student, but if we have this high divorce rate, what if we compare us to the national average?"

Carlo laughed. "You have a point. The divorce rate is growing everywhere and in every sector, unfortunately. According to Wilkinson and Finkbeiner (5), as of 2016, they reported:

1. Almost 50 percent of all marriages in the United States will end in divorce or separation.
2. Forty-one percent of all first marriages end in divorce.
3. Sixty percent of second marriages end in divorce.
4. Seventy-three percent of all third marriages end in divorce.
5. The United States has the sixth-highest divorce rate in the world.
6. Both marriage rates AND divorce rates in the US are decreasing.
7. The marriage rate in the United States is currently 6.8 per 1,000 total population.
8. The divorce rate in the US is 3.2 per 1,000 population (as of 2014, the last year of data from the CDC with 44 states

and DC reporting). This is known as the 'crude divorce rate.' Although useful for describing changes in divorce rates over time, the crude divorce rate does not provide accurate information on the percentage of first marriages that end in divorce."

He took a deep breath and continued. "According to the same group of lawyers (5),

1. Over almost 40 hours of work, 67 percent of first marriages terminate, more than the average.
2. Among all Americans 18 years of age or older, whether they have been married or not, 25 percent have gone through a marital split.
3. Fifteen percent of adult women in the United States are divorced or separated today, compared with less than one percent in 1920."
4. The average first marriage that ends in divorce lasts about eight years (3)."

13.4 Average First Marriage Duration

"Professions with the highest divorce rate:

- Dancers – 43%
- Bartenders – 38.4%
- Massage Therapists – 38.2%
- Gaming Cage Workers – 34.6%
- Gaming Service Workers – 31.3%
- Food and Tobacco Machine Operators – 29.7%
- Telephone Operators – 29.3%
- Textile Machine Operators – 29%
- Physician – 28.9%
- Nurse – 28.7%

As you notice, the physician is not in the top place, but they are running close to it," concluded Carlo.

"But doctor," Joyce asked again, "what can we do to avoid it and what can we do to not get there in the first place?"

"Well, Joyce, it is the same for all groups of physicians. Lack of commitment is the most common reason given by divorcing couples, according to a recent national survey. Here are the reasons that were given and their percentages:

- Lack of commitment – 73%
- Argue too much – 56%
- Infidelity – 55%"

"So, we should not be a doctor in the first place," commented Dr. Haney again. "Which profession should we take?"

"Well doctor," added Carlo, "the professions with the lowest divorce rates are:

- Medical scientists – 9.11%
- Other scientists – 8.79%
- Legislators – 8.74%
- Audiologists – 7.77%
- Dentists – 7.75%
- Farmers – 7.63%
- Podiatrists – 6.81%
- Clergy – 5.61%
- Optometrists – 4.01%
- Agricultural engineers – 1.78%"

"What about the financial effect to create the condition for divorce?"

"You are Dr. Metha, right? Well, the same group also answered other questions such as if finances affect the divorce rates; an annual income of over $50,000 can decrease the risk of divorce by as much as 30 percent versus those with a salary of under $25k. Feeling that one's spouse spent money foolishly increased the likelihood of divorce by 45 percent for both men and women. No offense to women; I summarized the article I took these data from."

13.5 Cost for the Taxpayers

The dean now was quite worried. "I am worried that you have scared our medical student!" he joked. "Tell me, is there a connection between the desire to divorce and moral distress syndrome and maybe suicide?"

Carlo was serious. He knew that it was hard data, and he felt sorry if he offended anyone. "Yes, there is a correlation," Carlo started with a leveled voice. "A new study entitled 'Divorce and Death' shows that broken marriages can kill at the same rate as smoking cigarettes. Indications are that the risk of dying is a full 23 percent higher among divorcées than married people. One researcher determined that a single divorce costs state and federal governments about $30,000, based on such things as the higher use of food stamps and public housing as well as increased bankruptcies and juvenile delinquency. The nation's 1.4 million divorces in 2002 are estimated to have cost the taxpayers more than $30 billion. An article in *The New York Times* stated that – of couples who seek marriage counseling – 38 percent end up divorced just two years later (3)."

References

1. R. Preidt. Doctors less likely to divorce, study finds. *Consumer*; 2015. https://consumer.healthday.com/public-health-information -30/divorce-news-204/doc.
2. Research Notes. *University Times*; 1997. https://www.utimes.pitt .edu/archives/?p=5326.
3. John Hopkins Medical Institutions. Physicians' divorce risk may be linked to specialty choice. 1997. http://articles.baltimoresun. com/1997-03-13/features/1997072018_1_divorce-rate.

4. Bruce L. Rollman, Lucy A. Mead, Nae-Yuh Wang, and Michael J. Klag. Medical specialty and the incidence of divorce. *The New England Journal of Medicine*; 1997; 336:800–803. https://www.nejm.org/doi/full/10.1056/NEJM199703133361112.
5. Wilkinson and Finkbeiner. Divorce facts and statistics. What affects divorce rates? 2017. http://www.wf-lawyers.com/divorce-statistics-and-fact.

Suggested Reading

D. P. Ly, S. A. Seabury, and A. B. Jena. Divorce among physicians and other healthcare professionals in the United States: Analysis of census survey data. *BMJ*; 2015; 350:h706. https://doi.org/10.1136/bmj.h706.

Emotional detachment. *Wikipedia*. https://en.wikipedia.org/wiki/Emotional_detachment.

E. E. Frezza. *The Health Care Collapse*. New York; Routledge; 2018; ISBN # 978-1-138-58110-4.

E. E. Frezza. *Tangled Sutures*. Austin, TX; TMA; 2018. www.texasmedicalassociation.org.

Doctors and stress. *The Federation of Medical Societies*. http://www.fmshk.org/database/articles/03mb1_3.pdf.

E. E. Frezza. *Medical Ethics*. New York; Routledge; 2018; ISBN # 978-1-138-58107-4.

S. Talbot and W. Dean. Physicians aren't 'burning out.' They're suffering from moral injury. https://www.statnews.com/2018/07/26/physicians-not-burning-out-they-are-suffering of moral injury.

E. E. Frezza. *The Miserable Doctor*. Sacramento, CA; Cure Your Practice Press; 2019; ISBN # 978-1-7047-7-3056.

E. E. Frezza. *Patient-Centered Healthcare*. New York; Routledge; 2019; ISBN # 978-0-367-14536-1.

Chapter 14

Medical Malpractice Insurance Crisis

In this session we will talk about:

- *Difficulties in obtaining malpractice insurance*
- *How malpractice insurance is obtained*
- *Premium increase*
- *The price of liability*
- *Is malpractice insurance mandatory?*

14.1 Difficulties in Obtaining Malpractice Insurance

"Doctor Bruni, I am Diana Klavan, the risk management director of this university. I have been having issues insuring new doctors lately, specifically, those who were in practice for a while. Lots of denial and inability to, therefore, hire the physicians. I have been looking into different companies, but it seems a losing battle. Do you know anything about this subject? What is going on?"

"I am not surprised to hear your question," replied Carlo. "Malpractice insurance is for-profit; they need to make money, and therefore, they try to avoid any high risk for them.

There are three specific problems in obtaining medical malpractice insurance:

1. Your application is evaluated by an entry-level secretary who is following a cooking book instruction; those administrators look at your age and number of claims you have and the state in which you like to practice.

2. Most of the insurance companies have a nonwritten rule: if you have more than three to five claims, you are out; they will not give you coverage. This is bad since they don't even read the claims, so if you win or lose the claims, you still lose the ability to have coverage, no questions asked. Nobody explains this rule or reason to you. You get to know this accidentally.

3. If you have an open claim, they don't consider the date the claim started, but when it was closed. Therefore, given the present legal system, if a claim takes eight years to close, the risk management teams at malpractice insurance companies consider that a new claim since the closing date for them is the starting date. This is totally unfair and unjust."

"Let me understand," replied Diane, "since in the USA anybody can sue anybody, there are many frivolous claims. Therefore, if you sue for frivolous claims, the insurance companies don't evaluate the consistency of the lawsuit, the merit, and the substance, but just a mere number?"

"Yes, you understand well. It does not matter the merit of the claim; it is all about the numbers. As you know, with all the patients looking to report things they don't like, even if they don't have medical substances, they always find a lawyer to represent them, and for these lawyers, there is no cost or repercussion to sue the doctor. Therefore, they can sue many times without any repercussions. Insurance takes advantage of the system by evaluating the mere number and not the merit of the suit.

In Europe, you can sue anybody, but if it has no substance or it is a frivolous suit, the sued party can actually countersue you. This decreases frivolous lawsuits. In the USA, the doctor cannot countersue the patients even if it was a silly claim. So, in the end, the doctor is 'screwed' twice!

Unfortunately, at the hospital level or at the university level, the risk management representatives don't know better and don't fight the medical insurance companies. They simply deny the hearing without explaining the situation to the doctor because they really don't know what to fight for or how to do it.

Unfortunately, I knew many physicians in this situation. I hope that you – being in charge of risk management – do your detective work. My friend was punished by denial of his full professorship and chairman position in Nashville, Tennessee, by the laziness and incompetence of the risk management director and the inability of the university to get out of their routine and think outside the box. He remained without a job for a few months. The pitiful thing is that both the dean and the president believed their risk management chair with-out looking into it. So, the question comes back again: who is defending the physician? It seems to me that the risk man-agement office plays against the physician in most hospitals instead of being the physician's advocate. After a few months, the dean was demoted and removed and the president did not do anything to amend the issue. It is too much work to defend and support a physician; it is better to let him go and take another one. Like you throw away a towel and you go to the shop and buy a new one. We physicians are becoming dispos-able objects in the hands of ludicrous people."

14.2 How Malpractice Insurance Is Obtained

The room was silent, and even Diane did not know what to say. Maybe she felt guilty, as many in her role should be.

Carlo then continued, "According to the American College of Physicians:

> Malpractice insurance is usually available through traditional insurance carriers or from a medical risk retention group, which is a mutual organization of medical professionals organized to provide liability insurance (sometimes sponsored by state medical societies). Additionally, some large medical systems may be "self-insured;" instead of purchasing commercial insurance, a medical liability trust fund is created that is used to pay for the defense of malpractice claims and any resulting judgments against their physicians. Although it is possible for smaller medical groups and practices to self-insure, there are significant legal and business obstacles that make this a difficult option for most.
>
> Individual and group malpractice coverage plans are available for those in independent or small practices. For employed physicians, medical liability coverage is typically offered as part of a group plan purchased by the employing hospital or health system. (1)"

14.3 Premium Increase

"It seems to me we are treated like car insurance: if you have an accident, it does not matter if it is your fault or the fault of the person who hit you. It is always your fault. Unbelievable! And your premium is going up, no questions asked.

According to Jean LeMasurier, who wrote about Medicare,

> Malpractice insurance premiums for physicians have increased at an average rate of over 30 percent per year. This rate is significantly higher than healthcare cost inflation and the increase in physician costs.

Trends indicate that malpractice related costs, both
liability insurance, and defensive medicine costs, will
continue to increase in the near future. Pressures to
limit physician costs under Medicare raise a concern
about how malpractice costs can be controlled. This
paper presents an overview of the problem, reviews
options that are available to policymakers, and dis-
cusses State and legislative efforts to address the issue.

Although malpractice costs may be a problem for
some physician specialties, overall the problem in
the short-term is limited. For Medicare, the problem
is less acute than for other health insurers because
less than 6 percent of Medicare costs for physicians'
services is spent for services from high-risk physicians such as obstetricians, neurological surgeons,
and thoracic surgeons. High defensive medicine costs
and the trend toward increasing malpractice premiums suggest that longer-term restructuring may be a
concern, particularly at the State level. (2)"

14.4 The Price of Liability

"William Sage (3) wrote,

> Liability insurance is typically priced according to the
> frequency and severity of paid claims associated with
> a physician's specialty and practice location (class
> rating). Physicians who perform risky surgery on
> younger patients whose legal damages are potentially
> significant (for example, orthopedists and neuro-
> surgeons), deliver babies who might suffer lifelong
> disability (for example, obstetricians), or diagnose
> life-threatening but potentially treatable diseases (for
> example, mammographers) pay much more for liabil-
> ity coverage than physicians who treat older patients,

avoid invasive procedures, or treat self-limiting ailments. These effects are magnified during crisis periods, as carriers abandon marginal markets and customers while applying increasingly conservative standards to physicians with whom they continue to do business.

Class rating is individually rational for insurers selling policies to large numbers of solo or small-group physicians but breaks down the ability of the healthcare system as a whole to reduce risk-bearing costs. Modern medicine is a collaborative enterprise; society gains nothing by discouraging physicians from entering high-liability fields such as obstetrics or neurosurgery. Neither does the current system offer meaningful incentives for specific physicians to improve safety; experience rating at the individual physician level is too imprecise to be effective. Finally, sharing liability costs to a greater degree among physicians (and other providers) would not threaten classic adverse selection against insurers because coverage is not voluntary. Although only a few states mandate that physicians carry malpractice insurance, hospitals and managed care organizations generally protect their own assets by obligating affiliated physicians to purchase such coverage. The only plausible justification for the class rating (and geographic classification), therefore, is based on fairness, not efficiency: Urban specialists often earn more than family practitioners in outlying areas. However, some lucrative specialties pay far less than others, and inner-city providers incur higher costs than their wealthier suburban counterparts.

According to the T. Baker study (4), the following specialties have the highest percentage of physicians with a malpractice claim annually, beginning with the highest risk specialty.

- Neurosurgery – 19%
- Thoracic-cardiovascular surgery – 19%
- General surgery – 15%
- Orthopedic surgery – 14%"

14.5 Is Malpractice Insurance Mandatory?

"No federal law requires doctors to carry medical malpractice insurance, but some states do. Whether or not doctors are required to have insurance depends upon the state where they practice. Roughly 32 states require no medical malpractice insurance and have no minimum carrying requirements, as Donovan Weger reported (5).

In the big picture, doctors don't have to have malpractice insurance. It is the hospital that requires insurance, so they can decrease their own liabilities. It is always easier to blame the physician for anything when it is convenient, as people often forget that without the physician, there is no hospital."

References

1. American College of Physicians. 2019. https://www.acponline .org.
2. Jean LeMasurier. Physician medical malpractice. *Health Care Financing Review.* 1985; 7(1):111–116. https://www.ncbi.nlm.nih. gov/pmc/articles/PMC4191514/.
3. William Sage. Medical liability: Beyond caps. *Health Affairs;* 2004; 23(4). https://www.healthaffairs.org/doi/full/10.1377/hlth aff.23.4.10.
4. T. Baker. Containing the promise of insurance: Adverse selection and risk classification. *Connecticut Insurance Law Journal.* 2002–2003; 9(2):371–396.
5. Donovan Weger. Going bare – are doctors required to have malpractice insurance? 2017. https://www.gallaghermalpractice .com/blog/post/going-bare-are-doctors-required-to-have-mal practice-insurance.

Suggested Reading

Michelle M. Mello, David M. Studdert, and Troyen A. Brennan. The new medical malpractice crisis. *The New England Journal of Medicine*. 2003; 348:2281–2284.

Kenneth E. Thorpe. The medical malpractice 'crisis': Recent trends and the impact of state tort reforms. *Health Affairs*; 2004; 23(1). https://www.healthaffairs.org/doi/full/10.1377/hlthaff.W4.20.

Frank Spencer. The malpractice crisis. *AMA Journal of Ethics*; 2005; 7(4):325–327. https://journalofethics.ama-assn.org/article/malpractice-crisis/2005-04.

https://www.medicaleconomics.com/news/abcs-malpractice-insurance.

David Belk and Paul Belk. The great American healthcare scam: How kickbacks, collusion and propaganda have exploded healthcare costs in the United States. Amazon; 2018. http://truecostofhealthcare.org/malpractice/.

E. E. Frezza. *The Health Care Collapse*. New York; Routledge; 2018; ISBN # 978-1-138-58110-4.

Chapter 15

The Opioid Crisis and Relief

In this session we will talk about:

- *The stress of prescribing opioids*
- *The opioid epidemic*
- *Expenditure on the opioid crisis*
- *Opioid abuse*
- *Physicians left alone with increasing patient demands*
- *The need for state and federal rules and a database*

15.1 The Stress of Prescribing Opioids

"Doctor, my name is Patricia Saxton, and I am an anesthesiologist working in the pain clinic. I have a lot of distress in my clinic with many people fighting to get opioids and treatments. Does this create stress and moral injury?"

"Absolutely," replied Carlo. "One of the most significant problems I see with how the evaluation system is used is in regard to pain relief. There are some patients who are quietly addicted to pain medications. They will complain about pain, no matter how much medication you prescribe. If you dare say anything to them other than 'Here's a prescription for what you asked for,' they will report you as a bad doctor. A few doctors have responded to this by being little more than drug pushers. That's not how I work."

15.2 The Opioid Epidemic

"The United States is experiencing an opioid overdose epidemic. Opioids (including prescription opioids, heroin, and fentanyl) killed more than 33,000 people in 2015, more than any year on record. Nearly half of all opioid overdose deaths involve a prescription opiate.

Drug overdose deaths and opioid-involved deaths continue to increase in the United States. The majority of drug overdose deaths (more than six out of ten) involve an opioid. Since 1999, the number of overdose deaths involving opioids (including prescription opioids and heroin) quadrupled. From 2000 to 2015, more than half a million people died from drug overdoses (1).

We now know that overdoses from prescription opioids are a driving factor in the 15-year increase in opioid overdose deaths. The number of prescription opioids sold to pharmacies, hospitals, and doctors' offices nearly quadrupled from 1999 to 2010. Yet, there has not been an overall change in the amount of pain that Americans reported. Deaths from prescription opioids – drugs like oxycodone, hydrocodone, and methadone – have more than quadrupled since 1999 (2, 3).

The most recent definitive data on the prevalence of the problem comes from the National Survey on Drug Abuse and Health, which surveyed 51,200 Americans in 2015. Based on weighted estimates, 92 million, or 37.8 percent, of American adults used prescription opioids in the previous year (2014); 11.5 million, or 4.7 percent, misused them and 1.9 million, or 0.8 percent, had a use disorder. The epidemic is spreading so rapidly that the numbers are likely higher now (4).

More than 140 Americans die every day from an opioid overdose, according to the Centers for Disease Control and Prevention.

In outlining its opioid plan, administration officials highlighted four areas. The plan allows expanded access to telemedicine services and giving doctors the ability to prescribe medications to treat addiction to those in remote locations. It speeds up the hiring process for medical professionals working on opioids. And it allows funds in programs for dislocated workers and people with HIV/AIDS to be used to treat their addictions.

In the Congress notes (5), the commissions set up to study the opioid crisis had to mandate educational initiatives at medical and dental schools to tighten opioid prescribing and fund a program to expand access to medications used to treat addictions."

15.3 Expenditure on the Opioid Crisis

"Congress is currently spending $500 million a year on addiction treatment programs, but that money runs out next year. The Trump administration says it will work with Congress on the budgeting process to find new money to fund addiction treatment programs. Recently, a group of Democratic senators introduced a bill that would provide more than $45 billion for opioid abuse prevention, surveillance, and treatment. Not coincidentally, that is the same amount of money Republican sponsors included for preventing opioid abuse in bills that would have repealed the Affordable Care Act.

Another option from the Congress notes would be to restore a funding cut proposed for the Substance Abuse and Mental Health Services Administration, the agency within the Department of Health and Human Services that oversees addiction treatment programs. In its 2018 budget, the Trump administration is proposing cutting the agency's budget by nearly $400 million (5)."

15.4 Opioid Abuse

"Opioid abuse rose dramatically between 1997 and 2007. There are a few points to make on the increasing number of chronic pain cases as follows.

1. The cost of chronic pain now exceeds that of cancer, diabetes, and heart disease combined in the USA
2. Fifty million Americans suffer from chronic pain
3. Seventy percent of these are undertreated
4. The US, with approximately 5% of the world's population, consumes 99% of the world's hydrocodone

Unfortunately, we are not ready to fight such a big battle, since physicians often struggle with ethical issues in pain management. Therefore, the undertreatment of pain has increased as both a public health problem and a human rights issue.

The physicians have been asked to be moral and legal gatekeepers in identifying legitimate pain patients. That started with medical school, although now the medical school curriculum rarely includes governmental regulation of pain management. For instance, 51 percent of Texas physicians believe prescribing long-acting opioids will lead to patient addiction.

From a survey done in 2011, Hambleton reported:

1. A decrease in prescription drug abuse in children and young adults
2. Only 19% of surveyed physicians received any medical school training in drug diversion and only 40% in substance use disorders (SUDs)
3. 43% of physicians do not ask about prescription drug abuse and diversion
4. 33% of physicians do not obtain old records before prescribing controlled substances
5. 66% of Texas family physicians are anxious about prescribing opioids for chronic pain (7)

Pain is the number one reason why patients visit medical facilities. Various approaches have been tried to encourage patients and physicians to talk about and allow for adequate treatment.

Every time a patient looks suspicious, they should be placed automatically in the database for controlled substances to prevent medicine shopping.

How we define a suspicious patient:

- Complain about excessive pain compared with clinical finding
- Take more medication than is needed
- Call office for more prescriptions
- A patient who does not pay for the visit

As physicians, we all should sign up for a database to follow up with our patients."

15.5 Physicians Left Alone with Increasing Patient Demands

"Physicians are an essential part of the solution to the epidemic of drug overdoses.

Nowadays, patients can write a blog about their physician on any medical web page. Unfortunately, unhappy patients use the internet to vent their frustration. Most of the time, their complaint is not legitimate.

This can negatively affect a physician's reputation online if only one unhappy patient complains and 1,000 other happy patients do not register their satisfaction. This is an entirely unfair system for the physician, which does not reflect the depth of their practice and their knowledge. A politician will be happy if 1 out of 100 voters is against them, but a physician cannot afford that.

Therefore, with an aggressive and challenging patient requiring pain medication, most of the time, the physician tends to give up and write a prescription because those patients are the ones reporting the physician who left them in pain. While instead, the patient should be informed of the opioid abuse. The health care system is not set up to help physicians defend against these abusive patients that can ruin their reputation. This increases doctor stress.

If healthcare providers aren't well, it's hard for them to heal the people for whom they are caring. Stress and burnout among practicing physicians may play a role in the opioid epidemic (7).

As burnout increases, satisfaction with work-life balance drops. Many physicians feel like they are playing a never-ending game. The answer to a growing cadre of masters: faceless managed-care bureaucrats, managers, IT consultants, quality measurement gurus, and the problematic patient is pretending more and more medications include opioids.

With scarce resources and the ethical duty to provide care for the patient, including assuring the patient that they have no pain and are healthy, the physician is then pushed to write the prescription.

Given these pressures and demands coming from so many quarters, some adult primary care physicians may not have enough time or the necessary emotional courage to explore non-opioid alternatives fully.

For example, when a patient with chronic lower back pain reports that 80 mg of oxycodone (OxyContin) per day has allowed him to continue working and providing for his family. Scenarios like this raise the possibility that physician burnout may be playing a role in the opioid epidemic (8)."

15.6 The Need for State and Federal Rules and a Database

"Having a database that can be shared between different pharmacies, hospitals, and doctors' offices is essential nowadays. Lots of patients in the past were 'doctor shopping' to get more drugs from a different office. Therefore, the database will completely solve this doctor shopping.

Another problem is when a patient gets different medicine from different doctors and then creates a homemade 'cocktail.' A database will provide evidence of 'cocktailing!' Therefore, we can eliminate noncompliance, 'do-it-yourselfers,' and prescription fraud."

References

1. NCHS. Drug overdose deaths in the United States, 1999–2016. NCHS Data Brief No. 294. 2017. https://www.cdc.gov/nchs/products/databriefs/db294.htm.
2. Z. Paster. Drug combos could pose a deadly threat. *Florida Times-Union*. 2017; August 9:E.1.
3. M. Serafini. The physicians' quandary with opioids: Chronic pain vs addiction. *NEJM Catalyst*; 2017. https://catalyst.nejm.org/quandary-opioids-chronic-pain-addiction/.
4. D. Noll. Landmark $270 million opioid lawsuit settlement opens door for dozens of pending cases. *Healio Rheumatology*; 2019. https://www.state.nj.us/health/populationhealth/opioid/opioid_deaths.shtm.
5. American Nurses Association. The opioid epidemic: The evolving role of nursing. 2018. https://www.ncsbn.org/2018_ANA_Opioid_Epidemic.pdf.
6. J. Achenbach, J. Wagner, and L. Bernstein. President Trump says opioid crisis is a national emergency, pledges more money and attention. *The Washington Post*; 2018. http://web.missouri.edu/~glaserr/3700s18/Opioids-topic/Emergency.pdf.
7. Hambleton 2013, *Morbidity and Mortality Weekly Report*. 49(23): June 28, 2010.
8. M/MMM. Gart. You're wrong. Pain is not a vital sign. *Kevin MD*; 2017. https://www.kevinmd.com/blog/2017/05/youre-wrong-pain-not-vital-sign.html.

THE DOCTOR, THE PERSON

2

Chapter 16

Training Hurdles

In this session we will talk about:

- *Foreign physicians*
- *The doctor and the man*
- *Getting a research fellowship*
- *Discrimination*

16.1 Foreign Physicians

"I think we are ready for a little coffee break before continuing; to stretch your legs," said Jeremy. "There was a lot of information, but we also want to know how Carlo became such an expert and what happened to him."

People stood up and stretched. Carlo was sipping his coffee. Most of the faculty came and shook his hand and complimented him for the amount of information he gave them.

When people came back, the dean said, "In truth, we were all here to hear the first part of your talk, but your information and your passion touched us so much that we are interested to know about your direct experience and how you dealt with that. For this reason, I asked every chairman to have their nurse practitioner and PA to start seeing patients while we can be here with you."

"I am honored and touched, sir," responded Carlo. "Let's make this less formal. Why don't you ask questions, and I will try to answer about my experience and other things you would like to know." The faculty heads and the resident nodded in full approval. They had started to like Carlo, and they wanted to know more.

16.2 The Doctor and the Man

"To start," said Mr. Diehl, "as a non-physician, I would like to know who you are as far as your family and how you got into the USA."

"The opportunity this great country gives to people. I am many things, but first, I am a man. After that, I am a surgeon. I am a scholar and academician. I am a businessman. Many times, I have been a defendant. The things I have been guilty of are not the things I have had to defend myself against.

My guilt lies in my relationships. I learned to rely on only myself at my father's knee. I learned that I could not rely on others since my school days. I learned that I didn't need others as I suffered through all sorts of social settings. From the playground to parties, I stood quietly trying to do my best and work hard and be me; I do not like those people that want to be better than you only by putting you down and not by working hard.

I tried hard to fit. My guilt was betrayal, but not in the classic sense. My deception was in not seeing what I had before it was too late. My betrayal was in failing to understand what others needed and expected of me. My deception is that I believed that others could be friends in the real sense of the words; I guess I am one of the least romantic (in the Latin meaning) in these words. Where friends are friends and foes are foes.

It was the parts of my life I had to defend, the parts of my life where I had no guilt or blame that taught me this.

I was born and raised in Italy to parents who grew up before and during World War Two. I was their only child.

My father was a very proud man who had been emotionally damaged in ways I have yet to understand fully. His emotional scars created loneliness in me that I didn't even begin to recognize until shortly before he passed away in 2016.

He was easily hurt. When someone offended my father, he would immediately forbid my mother or me from having anything to do with them ever again. My mother's family were some of his earliest transgressors. Looking back, it is clear that he felt threatened by them.

One thing my mother could do very well is keep a secret. She never lost her family, and he never knew that. I, however, grew up not knowing my aunts, uncles, and cousins.

In the earliest years of school, when kids are establishing pecking orders and teaching each other manners the hard way, I quickly established myself as a hard worker and multitasker; I wanted to be good. I was playing soccer, coaching basketball, working on private radio and TV, and writing for a local newspaper, and going to school. I did not have time for anything else. I was busy! I was healthy, secure. Later, in business, I realized that those social nuances very much apply to adults too. It was too late for me, though. I was characterized by my loner outlook, and I still am to this day.

Being smart and driven, and not being bothered by social expectations, I learned that I could accomplish anything I set my mind to. As long as I wasn't expected to be some social genius, I could do almost anything.

It was easy to respect me. I did what I said I would do. I achieved more than many of my peers. It was easy to overlook me too. I had no tolerance for fools or liars, and I still don't. Many social leaders are both. The one thing I have in common with those social leaders is loneliness.

When I decided to become a surgeon, nobody who knew me doubted that I could do it. It seemed reasonable for me to expect to become one of Europe's most excellent surgeons. Of course, reason in the mind of a 17-year-old is not reason, in retrospect, at over 50.

My inability to handle politics has always been my Achilles' heel. My refusal to play silly social games, to tolerate idiocy, corruption, lying, and self-deception did me no favors when it came to building my career. It didn't help my marriage either.

Padova University, in Northern Italy, has been teaching medicine since the 14th century. The school hosted Galileo Galilei, Nicolaus Copernicus, and William Harvey. Harvey was a British physician who was the first to accurately describe the circulatory system in 1628.

The university is still considered one of the most formidable in the world, with schools of law, science, economics, political science, medicine, and others.

After I got my degree there, I remained in Italy to do my first residency. But I had my eye on something more significant than being a hometown surgeon."

16.3 Getting a Research Fellowship

"I arrived in London, Ontario, in the summer of 1991 to meet Dr. Starzl, the man who had performed the first liver transplant and had a research team there; I wanted to work with them. During that trip, I also looked into a surgical position in the United States. I had then the pleasure to meet one of my first mentors; I still miss his direction and help nowadays when I moved away from transplant medicine.

I flew from Ontario to Minneapolis, Minnesota, to look into an opening for a colorectal surgeon. This was the work I had done in Italy.

Minneapolis was a beautiful city in the summer. The people were busily going about their lives as the Mississippi and

Minnesota rivers met and kept the area verdant and vibrant with the hustle of the people and the beauty of the land.

The meeting went well. I returned to Italy, hopeful. It was six months before I returned to America. I didn't go back to Ontario. I didn't go back to Minneapolis.

I moved to the USA with a research grant of $14,000 from Rotary International. Taxes ate half of that. All I could afford was rent, and for the first three months, I ate popcorn and peanuts with the occasional food from a nurse's party in the hospital. Then I learned about all-you-can-eat restaurants.

Legally, I was not allowed to work in the United States outside of the limitations of my research visa. Realistically, had I followed the letter of the law, my parents would have received my starved corpse within the year. I took what work I could for cash under the table. Mostly, I unloaded produce trucks. I was too proud to ask my parents for money!

I was working 18 hours a day and studying in the library. I was unloading fruit trucks every day, too, to get some bucks. Between the work and the lack of money to buy food, I lost 30 pounds in my first three months. I've never been a large man, and 30 pounds was significant for my build.

When my grant was up, nine months into my time there, the hospital started paying me $18,000 a year without benefits. I felt rich. I was finally able to pay for my exam, the board, and the English exams to get my MD recognized in the United States."

16.4 Discrimination

"These exams, as it turned out, were not run with the greatest of integrity.

We were assured that everyone took the same exam, and yet all immigrants had to take their exams in a different room. It reminded me of World War Two, but I have too much respect to mention what it really felt like and I will leave it to the reader's imagination! Later it was determined that our test was harder than the test given to the US graduates.

A life lived as a self-reliant loner helped me through that. My time at Padova and my endless studying paid off, and I passed despite the corrupt system. This was one time when my ignorance of political nuance probably served me. I thought something seemed off but didn't have the capacity or motivation to dig deeper into it, so I focused on the reason I was there, and I did well.

My father would not accept that I wanted to move to the United States to practice medicine. He told me many times that I would fail, go broke, and return home.

Because of this, no matter how bad times were, no matter how broke or hungry or sick I was, I stayed. I fought back. I kept moving forward.

My father came closer to being right than I ever let him know, and I kept doing whatever I had to do to be able to never ask for his help once I had arrived in the USA."

Chapter 17

Double Residencies

In this session we will talk about:

- *Double residency*
- *The pyramid system*

17.1 Double Residencies

"So, let me understand. You did the residency in surgery in Italy and then another one here? How is it possible? Was it easy to find a residency here?" asked Dr. Rothschild.

"Yes, I did, and unfortunately, it was not easy," replied Carlo. "I found a residency program in Washington, DC. I was there for one year after I sent 800 applications.

I was known as the 'White doctor' because I was the only one there who did not have African ancestry. For the most part, it was in good humor, and I got along well with the people there.

They also had a large contingent of Black immigrants from all over the world. It was interesting seeing the differences each culture had.

All in all, people were very kind. I didn't know how things worked in the United States, and they were accommodating. I had no problem with racism, gender issues, or anything like that, so I had a lot of fun with my peers.

From my first day, I tried to keep a low profile, as this Washington DC area was a high crime area.

I bought a car in Pittsburgh for $900 and drove it on duct tape and a promise until I got married. My first car cost me $300, so it was a step up.

Since I came to America as an adult, I had no history here. I didn't have credit, and insurance on a newer car would cost me $3,000 to $4,000. When I added my children onto my car insurance, it cost me £1,000, and they drove once in a while.

When I came in the 90s, they asked me for $2,500 for insurance. I learned that if you buy a car that is ten years old or older, you don't have to pay full coverage insurance; you can pay the liability. So, I bought a 15-year-old car, and my insurance was $300 a year.

I became very good at buying old cars. I have never purchased a new vehicle in the United States. Still, now, I buy a car for $300, $400, or $500, even though I am a doctor.

In those times, a lot of people wanted to be surgeons because it made a lot of money. At that time, a gallbladder surgery paid a surgeon $3,000. Now it pays $300. That's how much things have changed."

17.2 Pyramid Systems

"By my second year in the United States, I got a two-year preliminary residency contract in New Jersey. That was a pyramid set up.

In pyramid residencies, they start by hiring 20 young physicians. The schedule is grueling, up to 120 hours a week. The hospital is demanding beyond any good reason. The focus is on driving as many doctors out as they can. By the end of the program, they have three interns left. I was one of the three.

The theory behind this structure was that in a highly competitive atmosphere, only the best will come through. It was believed that such a system could create a higher quality medical community. In that, it failed.

The competition was so brutal that it kept young doctors from being able to collaborate successfully, to urge each other's genius to synthesize something better than any of them might imagine. The system treated humans as machines, and humans have proven we are not machines.

Pyramid residencies are no more after a major lawsuit.

After my third year, I finally saw the light with a contract for two years as a categorical fourth- and fifth-year resident in Staten Island, NY. I could finally finish my residency in the USA, and my hard work paid off. This is where I met your chairman, right, Jeremy?" Jeremy nodded. "I believe my self-reliance made all the difference for me in this corrosive system. I was able to excel because the things it required of me were my strengths. I was already a doer. I was already more comfortable doing than waiting. A go-getter they called me here in the USA."

Chapter 18

How Medicine Can Ruin a Marriage

In this session we will talk about:

- *Work overload and loss of family*
- *My first lawsuit and downfall*
- *Rebuilding yourself*
- *Travel and research*
- *Unnecessary suicide*

18.1 Work Overload and Loss of Family

"Over here, I am Geneva – a second-year family practice resident. I am an incurable romantic, so my question is: when did you get married? During the residency? And then did you do a fellowship?"

"Yes," replied Carlo. "I married and fathered my first son during the New York years. Finally, at almost 33, I was beginning my own family. This anchored me in a way that is still good for me over 20 years later.

Many doctors are so focused on their careers that their family becomes almost a distraction. Those doctors, in my opinion, would save themselves money and avoid many heartbreaks if they would create a family.

I knew that I could not be happy pursuing a career that left me bereft of family. It was time for a change.

My wife was my best friend, my consigliere. She is an academic, so we had great conversations about philosophy, academia, and life. We both have a strong love of family that made the time we shared with our boys some of the greatest memories either of us will ever have and still are!

I returned my growing family to Pennsylvania, where I began a transplant fellowship. It was at this time that my youngest and second son was born.

It didn't take long before I realized the demands of this fellowship weren't any better for a family man than those in New York had been. I slept in my bed, next to my wife, no more than three nights a month. I never had the time or energy to enjoy my life. I wanted a better and more strongly bonded family.

I started with the transplant fellowship, then I had an opportunity to switch to a laparoscopic fellowship with a focus on gastrointestinal and obesity, and I took that train. I finally started to see my family regularly and slept in my bed for more than 15 days a month!! It was too much work and responsibility to even think of having a family. Therefore, the laparoscopic fellowship looked very good!

When I went to my first job, I was the director of bariatrics. My chairman was sending his high-risk cases to me, and I was stupid enough to take them. This was the first time I got burned as a professional by a more senior professional."

18.2 My First Lawsuit and Downfall

"I did a surgery in October. I sent the patient home with wound care instructions. He didn't follow up with the nurse for wound care. He didn't show up to the office until he had an infection. We took the band out, and six weeks later, without me knowing anything more, he showed up in the hospital septic. I wanted to take care of him, but no surgery; otherwise, he would die in the OR. Unfortunately, the surgeon who took care of him took him to the OR, and he died. The family sued everybody but not the surgeon who took him to the OR.

When the patient was brought in for surgery, I told the on-call surgeon that he would die on the table. He was too weak. They needed to take some time to bring down the infection and build the patient's strength. They didn't listen to me. He died on the operating table.

The hospital was sued. Home health was sued. I was sued. What galls me to this day is that the hospital settled on my behalf without my consent.

After that, lawyers were attacking me from every direction like sharks after a wounded man. I had to leave for my sanity. I quit the hospital and returned to Pennsylvania. But my troubles were not over.

Sometime shortly after I had left that hospital, a patient came into the emergency room, and the clerk who did the intake put my name down as the attending physician. As a result, nobody saw the patient for three days, and he died.

Somehow, the family's lawyer decided that even though I was not employed there, and though my name was on the suit due to a clerical error, and even though I was working at a different hospital in another state, I should be held accountable for the patient's death.

That clerk's mistake and that lawyer's actions, be they via ineptitude or corruption, caused my malpractice premiums to suffer for 18 months while I fought to have my name cleared. The sharks were still looking for blood.

Back in Pittsburgh, I found a job, and I was taking calls also in a different hospital to make some extra bucks. During that time, alongside my surgical post, I worked in the emergency room and the intensive care unit to make ends meet."

18.3 Rebuilding Yourself

"Life was good in so many ways, but something was missing. Always, I was hungry to grow. While ambition should indeed be made of stern stuff, it can blind a man to what is right before him.

Then God gave me an appointment in Texas, and I was reborn, as was my mind, my body, and my ambition to be a good doctor and a good researcher.

I finally had room to expand and grow personally and professionally while still having time for my family.

I moved from Pennsylvania to Texas. At that time, I had a Volvo station wagon that I bought for $1,800 from an old lady. It took a day and a half to drive there. I stopped in a roadside motel that was so dirty I didn't want to sleep in it.

When I arrived in Texas – it was Father's Day – I unloaded everything I had into an efficiency apartment I had rented. I slept on an inflatable mattress for one year, waiting for my wife and kids to come and join me.

I arrived on Sunday night. I went in for my orientation on Monday morning. Everybody was very welcoming. I was shocked by how friendly and welcoming the people were in West Texas. Unfortunately, most people in town were not as open to someone with an accent. They found my accent amusing to the point of embarrassment. I often felt like a trained monkey when I'd hear, 'Say something!' Very few recognized that to me, they had the accents.

I bought a house and moved in by February, then all the furniture from Pittsburgh was sent down.

The years from 2003 to 2008 that we lived in Texas were the best years of my life. My wife and I were happy, and we had time to travel with the kids.

My family moved to Texas in June of 2003. My boys were aged six and three. I was beginning my new job as an assistant, and then I became an associate and then a full professor.

There I wrote 150 articles and 4 books; I was very productive. It's why I became a tenured professor so quickly.

With professionals, everything was okay. Outside of work was where things got tough for my children and me. I had to move my sons from a public school to a private school because of their Italian accent. I will always be grateful for the Christian school. They did a lot for my kids, and I will never forget them.

We started going to the swimming pool regularly. We went to basketball, volleyball, and football games; it was fun."

18.4 Travel and Research

"I was researching type II diabetes, hormone-based work that has since been completed by others. There are two pills on the market now that are based on the research I started. My trajectory was quite clear. I would start as an instructor of surgery and then assistant of surgery, an associate of surgery, then a full professor; I was tenured.

I was chief of minimally invasive surgery. Then I was chief of general surgery, and later I became the vice-chief of surgery and moved into a position where I could do research.

A group of researchers from China came to learn more about my work. They invited me to spend a few weeks teaching in China. I took my family, and my boys got to visit the Great Wall and spend time in Beijing while we were there.

I was invited to work in Japan. We took in Osaka, Yokohama, Tokyo, and Mount Fuji. When I was asked to speak in Greece, I took them to Athens and the Parthenon. During these years, I traveled the world lecturing. My boys visited their grandparents in Italy regularly.

Now, as young adults, I can see the foundation of worldliness these years have given them. I will always be grateful to have shown my boys a bigger world.

During my tenure, I earned my MBA (despite my wife's resistance!), published 4 books, wrote from 50 to 60 papers a year, and built my CV from 10 to 55 pages. A happy man can get a lot done. But sometimes, I wonder if, in my happiness, I was blinded to some conditions that led to my downfall.

These were the years that I was the only bariatric surgeon in Texas that covered New Mexico. I operated on many bariatric patients over those years."

18.5 Unnecessary Suicide

"I moved to this great new job and was in the process of changing. I reported to my new boss, and he already knew everything. I fully disclosed everything because I didn't want to have it thrown back in my face. I even told him about some new claims that would not be around for very long. Then one day, his boss called me. The office was populated by some professors, and they accused me of lying. The very thing I had protected myself against, the consequences of partial disclosure, was being thrown in my face. They accused me of lying. They refused to hear that I was in transition, that I had told my boss everything; all details were laid on the table from day one. They didn't have it. My preparation was for nothing. Their integrity was for nothing.

This man was on a crusade. My boss, the one I had disclosed everything to, committed suicide, and his boss had that covered up like it never happened. After running afoul of that man, perhaps I came out lucky only to lose my career. I suspect that, had he been out to get me, I would have lost more than I did, but to him, I was a disposable pawn. Isolating me as if I had the plague was all he needed to do.

The National Institutes of Health has only seven approved diabetic centers in the United States. I went to work in one of those.

I started the first week of August 2008 with a $1.5 million research grant to study possible cures for type II diabetes. A lab was ready for me to start my work.

The federal government announced its takeover of Fannie Mae and Freddie Mac on September 7 of that year. The subprime mortgage market was collapsing. A week later, major real estate investment firms started falling like dominoes. This was the real estate crash of 2008. My grant was tied to the market.

I was working on extracting a protein to create pills to cure type II diabetes. I lost my pills. I lost my patent. I lost everything. Those pills are now on the market, as another research team was able to continue the work.

We found a very nice two-bedroom apartment in a lovely neighborhood to live in. The kids went to a great school. I started working at a Veterans Affairs (VA) hospital as vice director of surgery. Losing the grant was frustrating, but I thought my career would remain stable, and my family was doing fine. I was still waiting for my university privileges. Then everything started falling apart.

The Wall Street Journal published an exposé about one of my bosses for inappropriate handling of VA funds. He went to jail. A few weeks after, my direct boss killed himself with a handgun, as mentioned earlier. He had attempted suicide a few times before, and his family thought they had him protected from his self-destructive urges. Unfortunately, they missed one credit card, which he used to purchase the gun. His wife found him in their house.

The hospital handled their part of the problem with a massive shakeup in personnel. I was among those shaken up with a blindfold over their eyes, and everybody was gone. But my boss was dead."

Chapter 19

The Legal Issues and Hollow Victory

In this session we will talk about:

- *Justice is blind*
- *Lawsuits kill souls*

19.1 Justice Is Blind

"It is quite a story," said Dr. Whittaker, the chair of trauma. "Now we are hungry for more. What happened next? The job was very grueling and then..."

The audience was silent and waited for more.

Carlo started slowly, "As it happens to highly paid professionals and insurance companies, I was the recipient of the occasional frivolous lawsuit. In Texas, I was sued even though I was not on call when the patient came in. The chair was on call. Nothing happened to him.

Justice is truly blind. Not only is she blind to the corrupting influences that might cause her to miscarry justice, but also to the corroding influences she often has on people's lives. More than two centuries of American court documents attest to the fact that justice must consider the well-being of the whole of society as more important than the welfare of the individual.

But sometimes, in those documents, you'll find that a person's life was ruined because a lawyer or a judge either dropped the ball or didn't give a damn. Officers of the court are human too. They get tired, overworked, and they burn out as quickly as anyone. There is recourse when justice fails someone. The problem is that it requires a drawn-out repeat of the process that just wore them down. By the time recourse is needed against injustice, the person who needs justice is emotionally exhausted and likely suffering financially or worse.

That's where I was when the Supreme Court finally decided in my favor, and the cases were closed. I had won. But I lost so many things on the way that it is just painful to remember. That was one hollow victory, empty as the space around me! I kept sitting and closing my eyes. My life ran like a fast-paced movie; I started filling the 'hollow' with memories, pain, and 'sorrow'!"

"What happened? What cases?" said the Dean. "I did not hear any cases."

"Yes, because you are on the east coast. This was a Midwest case that became so convoluted that it required a Supreme Court ruling."

"Can you tell us about it?" Mr. Diehl asked, "or is it still under investigation?"

"This patient went to a doctor who did not understand these convoluted issues, did not research it, and did not call me to ask about my previous work on his patient. He told her and others they needed to have the surgery done over, but he was wrong. They needed a simple endoscopic procedure, and still, today, after they have sued me, they don't know about it."

19.2 Lawsuits Kill Souls

"This was a defining moment for me. I was accused thanks to the ignorance of someone else! I had been operating on the premise that doing my work conscientiously, accountably, and professionally would leave me untouched by any severe malpractice claims. I knew there would be frivolous claims; society has been lawsuit-happy for a long time now.

What I learned the hard way, is that a combination of stubborn refusal to self-educate on the part of another doctor and a lawyer could be enough to bring me down. The legal system is not without culpability, either. Although the decision of the Supreme Court was technically in my favor, I now have permanent damage done to my reputation. I have lost my family, much of my career, and countless hundreds of thousands of dollars in income.

The nine years this attorney spent attempting to sue me wasted his time. It consumed his client's time and money. It wasted my time, money, and the most significant parts of my life. Had he studied a bit before deciding to sue, he probably never would have tried this. He sued the wrong doctor. The other surgeon did the incorrect operation. He should fix the issues with a simple endoscopic procedure, but he did not know better. He was the one to blame.

Between the surgeon and the lawyer, it was determined that I already had the plague. I had been the recipient of enough stupid lawsuits that I looked like an easy mark. I most definitely was not an easy mark. I regret what happened to me. I hate what happened to the sick patient; she was a pawn in their game.

Texas requires a qualified medical professional written report before a malpractice suit can be filed. New Mexico does not. While New Mexico does need a medical expert to testify in some cases, there are no restrictions upon that professional witness. That leaves room for an attorney to paint a beautiful picture. Until the end, the plaintiff's attorney kept pushing my attorney to settle out of court. Everybody knew it wouldn't be much longer before the case was finally decided. Perhaps he knew he was going to lose; I don't know. What I am sure of is that he chose me as an 'easy target,' and he ramped up his efforts to get an out-of-court settlement toward the end.

My hollow victory was empty, cold! I felt misery descending on me! I touched the bottom by winning! This was a kind of horror movie experience. I felt like I could not talk, I could not speak for many years. 'Dead men tell no tales' as in the *Pirates of the Caribbean* movie. Me, the ghost, will always remain a ghost, because if he comes back to life, he will die again!"

"It is unbelievable," the crowd said.

"How can we be more protected from legal injustice?" commented Dr. Whittaker. "As a trauma surgeon, we see many problems that need to be fixed ASAP, and then after a few years, the lawyer tells what we should have done. I guess it is always easy to be the quarterback the day after, but when the ball is hot in your hand, you have to make a decision, and that is why there are not too many good quarterbacks."

Chapter 20

Inability to Return to Work: The Apex of Moral Distress

In this session we will talk about:

- *Challenging yourself: the paranoia*
- *Second-guessing*
- *Fibrin or pus?*
- *Your CV is not good anymore*

20.1 Challenging Yourself: The Paranoia

"How difficult was it to return to work or to work with all the things on your mind? This must be the apex of the moral distress a surgeon can go through," asked Jeremy, the chair of surgery.

"Guilty until proven innocent! That's what it feels like to be accused of something in this country. No, I didn't go to jail, but if I had honestly been seen as innocent, I wouldn't have lost everything I'd built up either. Guilty until proven innocent is heavily flawed. Everybody looks at me like I'm a criminal. It doesn't matter if the problem is someone else's. It doesn't matter if the accusation is false. It doesn't even matter if the charge isn't all that damning. Once people start looking at you like you're a pariah, you're a pariah. Sometimes I think I could have committed murder and been treated better.

Everybody was talking about me. Nobody was talking to me unless it was to ask embarrassing questions. In a committee meeting, I'd get looked at with disdain, and I could read the question on their faces, 'Why is he sitting on a committee that I'm on,' as though I was carrying a contagious disease. I was already depressed. I had considered suicide. I couldn't go to my colleagues for mental health treatment; they thought I was guilty too. It's hard to go back to work under such conditions.

I found myself second-guessing everything I did. I was always looking over my shoulder to see if trouble was coming. My blood pressure went up, and I've been on blood pressure medication since. I have become extra careful with what I say to patients, the nurses, the secretaries, and, of course, other physicians. Even a harmless comment can become damning evidence of some imagined infraction. You don't want any more problems. You don't want comments. You don't wish to gossip. You want to do your job and get out. Every day at work was like running the gauntlet. Sometimes a patient would make a comment that would catch my attention, and I would begin to fear to treat that patient. It is a fear that is hard to describe. It seems to filter up from the bone marrow and encase me in hardened calcium. I'm sure those who have been on the receiving end of a lawsuit know what I'm going through. I don't necessarily think everyone is out to get me, so I'm not paranoid. I think everyone is feeding the rumor mill, and that will bring me down. They're not malicious; they're just careless. There's no comfort in the difference."

20.2 Second-Guessing

"I would be in surgery, performing an operation I had done 3,000 times. I would put in a stitch that was not text-book perfect and think, 'I hope nobody saw that.' Then I start doubting if I should even be doing surgery. From there, I started questioning if I should be in public at all. All this pain and fear over a surgery that I performed excellently.

I wasn't the only one second-guessing myself. My patients would come to me after seeing their primary care physician and tell me that I hadn't given them enough pain medications or antibiotics. I give antibiotics according to the accurate indication. I give pain meds according to reasonable need.

A patient expects to leave the office with a prescription. They come in one time, and you give them a script for Bacitracin. They come in another time, and you provide them with a script for antibiotics. They come in another time; you provide them with a prescription for pain medication. If they come back again, you can give them medicine for a chocolate bar, and they'll be happy. When you're more concerned about what they say about you than you are about doing your job right, it's time to step back and reevaluate a few things.

It's interesting how often a nurse, nurse practitioner, a physician, and others will say that a wound is infected when it isn't. That is why there are so many infections resistant to antibiotics. We prescribe antibiotics like water! As soon as a patient goes to see somebody else, the wound is automatically infected. Ask those same people the difference between pus and fibrin, and they'll look at you like you're from Mars. If you're going to diagnose an infected wound, first learn what fibrin is.

Fibrin is white, like pus, but unlike pus, it is not a liquid. It is an insoluble protein formed during the clotting of blood, which impedes the flow of blood. In other words, fibrin is good, is necessary, and is not going to go away due to antibiotic use."

20.3 Fibrin or Pus?

"It is common for a surgical wound to be a little bit open at first, and fibrin will be evident. So many practitioners see it as pus without bothering to check. All they need to do is take a sterile Q-tip and touch the white stuff. If it breaks down, it's pus. If it doesn't break down, it's fibrin, and that means that the wound is healing correctly and is not infected.

The first time a patient sees the fibrin, they panic. They run to their primary care physician (PCP), and he prescribes Bacitracin to calm them, knowing full well there's nothing wrong. Or worse, he prescribes it thinking it's enough to fix an infected surgical wound. It wouldn't be much trouble for the PCP to tell the patient, 'that is not an infection you're looking at, it's fibrin, and it's a good sign that you're healing well.' But the patient is panicking, and they're putting on the pressure, and the PCP is already stressed enough, and he knows they'll go away happy. We spend entirely too much energy and time worrying about how our patients are going to talk about us. Getting a sound report card from a patient is often more important than educating them. God save us.

I have found one way to help people remember the difference between fibrin and pus. It helps them avoid some high-calorie foods, too, so, for my bariatric patients, this is a double win. If you like Boston cream, think about its texture and color. It is the same as pus. It will break down when you touch it with a fork/Q-tip. I may single-handedly ruin the popularity of Boston cream." The audience laughs. "It is like having bubonic plague." Carlo was trying to make a joke.

"During the bubonic plague in Europe, affected people were moved to remote locations, such as highlands and mountains, far away from society. Most died in those locales, of course, but the idea was that they would not spread their incurable disease to everyone else. The plague is now better understood, and there are medical responses available. Isolation is no longer necessary."

20.4 Your CV Is Not Good Anymore

"Where isolation seems necessary is in litigation. There's no cure for becoming a defendant outside of 'good old boy' repackaging, which is in limited supply. I get told, 'Hey, your CV is great, but no thanks' and 'Hey, you have more experience than we require, but no thanks.' There is no explanation. Those claims are the plague. Isolation is my lost life.

It's interesting to note that in the eight years that I have been performing surgeries in small hospitals, some even owned by large corporations, nobody has filed a lawsuit against me. When I consider that none of the previous lawsuits had made a legitimate claim against me, and the rather high number of them, it's easy to feel as if someone wanted me out of the way, or perhaps I was just an easy target being a loner immigrant working in high dollar institutions.

None of that matters, though. I still have the plague, regardless of how I got it. Economically, this cost me eight years' salary as a professor in chief. It cost me moving money many times over, and it cost me lost pension contributions. In reallife, the cost of the intangible and invaluable losses was far higher. Before this, I had been popular in the meeting and research circuit. I was always invited and always traveling to meet new people. I had my hotel and flights covered. I had a genuine chance of discovering a drug to cure type II diabetes, but of course, the plague ended my research. There is no value that can be placed on all of that I was kept from doing. It is the value of family. It is the value of improving millions of lives. It is the value of fulfillment. It is truly priceless."

Suggested Reading

Ann Marie Corrado and Monica L. Molinaro. Moral distress in health care professionals. *University Western Ontario Medical Journal*; 2017; 86(2). http://www.uwomj.com/wp-content/uploads/2017/12/vol86no2_12.pdf.

Edwin Leap. Once upon a time being a doctor was great. Not anymore. 2017. https://www.kevinmd.com/blog/2017/02/upon-time-doctor-great-not-anymore.html.

Will people have a personal physician anymore? *Can Fam Physician*; 2017; 63(12):909–912. https://www.ncbi.nlm.nih.gov/pmc/articles/PMC5729133/

SOCIETY AND THE SUFFERING PHYSICIAN

Chapter 21

Societal Responsibilities

In this session we will talk about:

- *Tort reform and safe tax dollars*
- *Societal responsibilities*
- *Unhappy patients write bad reports, happy patients don't write*

21.1 Tort Reform and Safe Tax Dollars

"Hello – I am Mr. Johnston – I am the legal counsel for the University, and your story strikes me. Is the legal environment that bad? Did you learn some from this legal mess?"

Carlo thought for a moment and said:

"I understand that being just one person in a more significant situation, my needs are my responsibility. I also appreciate that this more significant situation cost a great deal more people than just me. Tax dollars were spent on this paying the judge and court employees to pursue something that should never have been on their desks. Plaintiffs lost time and money coming after me only to learn I was innocent. Did they have the motivation to sue those responsible later, or like me, are they so emotionally spent that they can't even think about going back into a courtroom? There is a resource for tort attorneys of experienced jurists who comment on the advisability of a lawsuit before any claims are filed. I have to wonder if the attorney made use of that resource. Did the attorney have all the information? When he found out that I could prove that I could not possibly be culpable for this claim, was it too late for him to change, or was he merely not motivated? I'll never know.

Living in this society has been a challenge for me. I've had to adapt to many things. Some I didn't even know existed. I didn't know about Medicaid before I moved here. I didn't realize the entitlement that many on Medicaid have. I'm not saying they don't deserve care. I am saying that my tax dollars are paying for their care, so I want them to use it wisely and take care of themselves."

21.2 Societal Responsibilities

"I've noticed that people have a bunch of ready excuses for why they're so sick. They also make plans and promote themselves, and sometimes others, that they're going to change their behavior. It's not my job to stay home with them and tell them what to eat. It's not my place to go grocery shopping with them. It's my job to help them change their health for the better, but I am only one part of a more abundant life-changing program.

That program is an uphill battle. Society, advertising, and even television shows normalize lousy eating habits, smoking, and drug habits. Of course, when you interview them they don't smoke and don't drink and don't do drugs. They always lie to you.

Making changes requires taking significant responsibility. To make that kind of trust, a person has to find a way to get comfortable with it, and that isn't easy. Nobody must take responsibility for themselves; it is optional. But to abdicate one's duty and then expect others to pay the consequences is dishonest. It's common too.

When I was teaching, I graded a student's work as I was somewhat capable. I was amazed at how many who earned a C would fight me to change it to an A. I would tell them if they had put the energy they're using to fight the C they earned into studying, they would have received an A.

They would get their revenge after the course was over by filling in a report card with the school. Those report cards go to the dean. If you get enough bad grades, as a teacher, you lose your job. Many professors teach to the report card and not to the student's learning.

The result is a reinforcement of the system of unearned entitlement. The result is the society of pseudo-professionals who cannot perform their jobs adequately because they are afraid of failure. I don't want to go under that surgeon's knife!

A good teacher should have no reason to fear a few complaints. He should know that the school has discerned that he is worthy of their support through continued impartial assessments. This is the only hope we have for training the next generation of professionals."

21.3 Unhappy Patients Write Bad Reports, Happy Patients Don't Write

"This report card system, which is a part of post-evaluation questionnaires after the patient's visit, can be dangerous. Only the unhappy patients write a report, and the happy ones tend to forget about it. The patient gives a scorecard to the hospital, grading their doctors on their work. If this were seen as part of a more extensive assessment system, and if it were used primarily to seek out patterns in doctor-patient relationships that might need to be addressed, or encouraged, this could be a good thing. Instead, it is used by corporate heads to lop off the professional heads they deem unnecessary or threats.

Unhappy patients always write a report, but happy patients don't, and this situation has skewed the data toward adverse reports. Therefore, data taken from the web or Press Ganey data are wrong because they report data with a standard deviation too significant to be considered. If those data were statistical analyses, they would not even be considered since they are five to six times away from the bell curve. But in healthcare, they do. They need 15 to 18 percent of patient reports to make a number, and with that number, they deny your bonus or promotion.

Unfortunately, everybody looks at the report but nobody look at the number of patients you treat, which makes one complaint a minuscule number. Maybe we should use some math, and compare the fraction of bad reports to the total number of patients you have treated, and not focus on one or two reports. For instance, if I have two bad reports over 5,000 patients, two divided by 5,000 is 0.04 percent of my patients! That is very good and not very bad as they try to depict you.

I was working for a new healthcare company that started using scorecards for the patients to evaluate their care. The company has an intranet where only employees can see what's posted. I could go there and learn how many patients were complaining about me and how many were happy with me.

This was in south Texas, where 75 percent of the people don't speak English well. Most of the comments were in Spanish. The designers of the web page hadn't considered the language differences, so those who had little to no English had to guess what the questions said or ask someone to translate for them.

There was a far bigger problem, however. On my report card that was available for everyone to see, I had four bad comments. These four bad comments seemed to be sufficient to worry the CEO and others in management. They didn't bother me because I can do the math.

I had 1,600 cases at that time. I had seen 5,000 patients during that same time. I had performed 800 surgeries, also during that time. So, my disapproval rating was just under 1 per 1,000 (less than 1 percent!). If I were running for President of the United States with a 99 percent approval rating, I'd be the most popular president in history.

I'm pretty sure those managers could do the math as well. They weren't punishing me because I had a meager disapproval rating. They were panicking that someone didn't like their system. They also used it as an excuse not to pay me the bonus they had promised me.

People who are happy with your work seldom take the time to respond to evaluation requests. It's the people motivated by anger, frustration, and fear who seek out the opportunity to lambaste someone who served them. Indeed, some bad reviews were earned. I might have received one or two in my career. But if every patient I worked with evaluated my work, I'd be the surgeon general by now."

Suggested Reading

Patients responsibility code from AMA. *Code of Medical Ethics*; 2017. https://www.ama-assn.org/delivering-care/ethics/patient-respon sibilities.

Patients responsibilities and right. *HHS*. https://www.hhs.gov/answe rs/health-care/what-are-my-health-care-rights/index.html.

Physician responsibilities by AMA. *Code of Medical Ethics*; 2017. https://www.ama-assn.org/sites/ama-assn.org/files/corp/media -browser/code-of-medical-ethics-chapter-1.pdf.

Chapter 22

Emotional Detachment and Patients' Responsibilities

In this session we will talk about:

- *Emotional detachment*
- *Patients need to give full disclosure*

22.1 Emotional Detachment

"Hello, over here." A white-haired senior doctor was waving. "I am Dr. Burke, an old internist. I did see in my many years of practice, a change in the attitude of the patient and also of the doctors. What do you think are the responsibilities of a doctor and the patient? If there are any?" he said, shaking his head.

Carlo thought for a moment and then said, "One of the highest responsibilities a doctor can have, that is not often considered, is emotional detachment.

Emotional detachment is a learned skill. To stand in the face of risk, trauma, or tragedy and keep a cool head requires a degree of detachment. Once learned, it can be achieved with a simple decision, not unlike flipping a switch. Some professions require this skill to varying degrees. Doctors and especially surgeons, need to develop it to a very high degree.

A person who can effectively utilize emotional detachment can set evident boundaries. Be it in social situations, during family strife, or in their professional discernment, these people earn great respect for their ability to remain calm and make clear decisions, all the while respecting the emotions of others. For the majority of people, emotional detachment is a far cry from reality. Choosing not to engage when emotions run high seems impossible to most people. Unfortunately, the news media, entertainment sources, politics, and even religious leaders can feed this disempowering lie. Emotional detachment includes empathy. Without empathy, emotional detachment would be cruel. There is a common myth that compassion requires vulnerability. It is only through honest emotional detachment that one can be of service with empathy.

This is the balance a doctor strives for every day. Whether we must give a patient bad news, or we are helping them come to an informed decision from an emotionally charged place, we must first empathize, and then we must detach. A doctor must learn emotional detachment, and he must own it completely. Any doctor can find himself in the face of shocking trauma at any time; it's one of the characteristics of the profession. This is a large part of why doctors often have an air of authority and are often seen as wise.

Emotional detachment in empathy allows one space to rationally choose their responses without being drawn into a state of being overwhelmed or manipulated. Emotional boundary management is an effective and universal tool. Whether responding to an overwrought patient or an overwhelmed peer, the management of emotional boundaries is crucial to maintaining one's integrity, dignity, and choice capacity.

There is almost a mystique around a self-possessed, emotionally detached person. The skill is so rare as to inspire awe in many. The simple act (once learned) of deciding to step aside from current drama is powerful. Anyone can learn it, but few realize this."

22.2 Patients Need to Give Full Disclosure

"Just as a doctor must maintain healthy emotional boundaries of empathy and detachment, the patient must fully and honestly disclose everything about their life that might in any way contribute to the problem they are seeing the doctor about.

So many activities that harm the body or foster disease are illegal, or at the very least, they inspire social censure. Drug use, unsafe and promiscuous sexual practices, binge eating, or binging and purging are standard practices over which people fear being judged.

These subjects should be part of the very first consultation between doctor and patient if the doctor is going to give the patient their best chance at healing. This is another crucial time for a doctor to strike that balance between empathy and detachment. If a patient feels judged for their behavior, they will not fully open up, and the doctor will not be sufficiently informed to help them.

Some patients will take the opposite viewpoint. They willfully disclose every striking thing to their doctor knowing that should the doctor evince judgment, they can call him on it; and should the doctor break confidentiality, they can sue him. These patients are often angry, and a degree of calming influence is needed on the doctor's part along with evident empathy, detachment, and a willingness to speak frankly with the patient on their level.

The patient needs to know they have a voice with their doctor.

They need to know that the doctor is taking the time to understand them fully. They need to see the doctor is taking them seriously, especially when they expect to be dismissed. In short, the patient must feel safe to disclose everything the doctor needs to know to help them."

Suggested Reading

A. Kerasidou and R. Horn. Making space for empathy: Supporting doctors in the emotional labour of clinical care. *BMC Medical Ethics*; 2016; 17:8. doi:10.1186/s12910-016-0091-7.

Emotionally detached concern or empathic care. In: *Humanizing Modern Medicine. Philosophy and Medicine*, Dordrecht; Springer; 2008; 259–276.

Chapter 23

Do Patients Want to Participate in Their Care?

In this session we will talk about:

- *How patients have no rules*
- *Why we need professional patients*
- *Physician-centered healthcare*

23.1 Patients Have No Rules

"I tend to agree with you – I am Darren Rothgery, vice-chair of family medicine – patients' lack of ownership in their health is the trademark of US healthcare. When people are sick, they go to the hospital; in the meantime, they can do what they like, smoke, drink, gain 200 pounds above your supposed healthy weight. This is a system that resuscitates patients! But you cannot be revived at all. If you are sick, you are ill, and if you did not take care of yourself for years, maybe nothing can be done for you."

"I share the same feeling," said Traci King from family medicine. "What has been lacking is a plan and a strategy to teach patients to care for themselves as much as possible. In countries with a social system, the patient doesn't go to the emergency room unless it is necessary; they have a physician to call instead. Patients try to modify their diet, smoking habits, etc. to be more healthy.

A chronic disease like diabetes, emphysema, arthritis secondary to being overweight, etc. can be cured with better patient education."

Carlo then concluded, "More critical though, we need to work the basics as well by training new patients into a better and healthy life and into more self-conscious self-care. They need an understanding of what they have to do to achieve it and protocols and policies to sustain a better life.

Prevention has always been the pinnacle of any medical care and should be brought back as a base upon which to build new healthcare for the next century."

He took a deep breath and continued, "The medical field was based on the trust the patient placed on the physician to make the right decision. It is defined as a 'paternalistic system' (4). Nowadays, the pendulum is changing; there are no more patients listening to their doctors; patients want and need to participate. It is not more ordering and advising the patient, but a conversation with the patient about the order and advising on plans and treatments available.

It is like a more round-table approach where the patients are informed and trust the physicians to suggest the right options.

When we were young, we were going to the physician and only listening to options; now we talk and listen to our options. That means that the patient can also ask a question, and they are welcome to ask questions. At the same time, though, the same patient thinks they know more since they read it on the internet. We advise against this as there is so much information on the internet, and some of it is written by nonexperts in the field. These people do not have the background and the knowledge to publish their video or their advice and create only problems by creating confusion.

Therefore, we need to encourage patients to be proactive about their health within the context of this provider/patient relationship. However, we still encourage patients to listen only to the experts and not the 'Monday morning quarterback.'

It will be fantastic to create and share documentation, share decision making, common goals, and treatment that patients and families share and agree upon, like having a contract to purchase a house. Possible complications and side effects of lacking medical care should be shared with the patient.

The problem that we face is that patients do not like responsibility and put all the blame for their care on the physician. Most of the patients I got in contact with don't want liabilities, so if something goes wrong, they can blame or sue the physician.

This is too easy because their health starts with them, and if they do not do anything to fix themselves, the physician does not have a magic ball to cure them. At the same time, the physician can definitely be more successful if their patients are compliant.

This sharing view starts with patient compliance, and that is difficult to find. Why does healthcare always blame the physician? The patients' lack of responsibility should not be penalizing physicians when the patients themselves do not follow their treatment plan."

23.2 We Need Professional Patients

"I am Veronica Paez, a first-year resident in medicine. I went to medical school to help people, and now I find I am defending myself from them. Is this possible? Why do we need to be careful of the people we are supposed to be taking care of? How can we solve this puzzle?"

Carlo answered, "If the physician will welcome feedback, the patient has to do the same, and not just write an ugly criticism about the physician on the web because they can! It is not possible to have a shared vision with patients who cancel their visit at the last minute; otherwise, the system will fail. Those patients do not care that the time in the clinic allotted for them can be used for someone else who needs to see the physician that day. They don't care about others as they do not care about the physician. If they do not buy the medications, get the appropriate workup, do their x-ray, etc., they suffer no consequences whatsoever. But if we physicians don't do one little thing we get sued.

These situations place even more stress on physicians to share their plans. They need to involve the patient, they need to do many things, but they do not have a counterpart, the patient, who will work with them. The physician deserves a better partner in professional patients, not just patients. Those that don't want to be professionals should not seek advice since they know they will not follow through with it. There are many consequences physicians will suffer if they don't do their job, but none for patients. The patient needs to be held accountable and reported to their health insurance, which can decide if it wants to cover them or not.

If you book a hotel and you do not go, you lose your deposit; the patient does not lose anything except their health. Patients need to be responsible for themselves and others since if they don't show up to the office, they take a spot from somebody else who is waiting. If they canceled a surgery the night before, they take precious time from another human being that might need the surgery more than them.

This shows a complete lack of care for themselves and the society they live in. Unfortunately, nowadays, health-care and everyone, administration first, are catering to these patients, and no one wants to say anything bad to them, which is wrong since we are perpetuating a negative attitude and situation that affects the lives of other human beings. We need to put a stop to it and make patients take their own responsibility, because miracles do not happen if they don't take care of themselves."

The dean intervened, "If we want patient-centered care to work, we need to have patients be professional as well and not forget about their health, forget to do their labs and tests simply because they 'forget.' Forgetful patients need to be educated, and if the forgetfulness persists, they need to suffer the consequences and be fired as a patient and have a member of their healthcare insurance informed because they are a liability not to the system, but overall, to themselves.

We are in a democratic country; they can do whatever they want, but they cannot come back and blame others for their forgetfulness. Let's stop this madness and get healthcare back in shape."

Everybody applauded.

23.3 Physician-Centered Healthcare

Carlo then added, "Too many people have forgotten that besides the patients, also the physician and the provider are the customers of healthcare; without them, healthcare would not exist.

If we take all the administrators out of the hospital, it will be business as usual, but if you take out physicians and nurses, the hospital will close asap.

So, it is time to see the patients and physicians as customers, and to have a sense of why we wake up in the morning and do this job to help providers give healthcare to others. Patients deserve happy physicians.

We always talk about patient-centered healthcare, to make it easy for the patients, but nobody has defined what makes it more accessible for the physicians. Maybe we should think about physician-centered healthcare for once" (1).

"I am Rocio Menchaca. I am a pediatrician, and I am tired of the abuse of patients coming to the office, refusing vaccinations, and refusing to sign a form produced by the American Association of Pediatrics where they take responsibility for their refusal. Then we are liable. One of the common problems nowadays is the refusal to vaccinate. Society accepts this even if it is a risky enterprise. Now, if you refuse something for your children, you take responsibility for it. But parents are refusing to sign the refusal form. They don't want the vaccine, but if something goes wrong, they want to sue the physician for not having given the vaccine. This happened to a pediatrician in the last two years where they got sued and found guilty. Now pediatricians don't want to see those parents and kids. Do you blame them? We don't want to be like our colleague; he lost the case because the parents did not understand that the child could die if they were not vaccinated! Where is common sense?"

The crowd applauded.

Reference

1. Charles W. Smith, Terry Graedon, Joe Graedon, and John Grohol. A model for the future of health care. *Society for Participation Medicine*; 2013; 5:20.

Suggested Reading

E. E. Frezza. *Tangled Sutures*. Austin TX; TMA; 2018. www.texasmedicalassociation.org.

J. G. W. S. Wong. Doctors and stress – The Federation of Medical Societies. *Medical Bulletin;* 2008; 13(6). http://www.fmshk.org/database/articles/03mb1_3.pdf.

E. E. Frezza. *Medical Ethics*. New York; Routledge; 2018; ISBN # 978-1-138-58107-4.

E. E. Frezza. *The Miserable Doctor*. Sacramento, CA; Cure Your Practice Press; 2019; ISBN # 978-1-7047-7-3056.

E. E. Frezza. *Patient-Centered Healthcare*. New York; Routledge; 2019; ISBN # 978-0-367-14536-1.

Chapter 24

It Is Challenging to Be a Physician

In this session we will talk about:

- *How physicians like to be physicians*
- *The high standards we have to follow*
- *Decreased reimbursement and more responsibilities*
- *Difficulties being a surgeon and making decisions in seconds*

24.1 Physicians Like to Be Physicians

"After all of these bad experiences and dealing with difficult patients, do you still like being a surgeon?" asked the chair of medicine.

"I would not do anything else," answered Carlo. "It's gratifying to apply my training and experience in the face of a complex medical problem and figure out what's wrong. When I work hard in the operating room to repair damaged tissue or to help set a patient on the path to a healthier future, it fulfills me. More than that, I genuinely like what I do, and that is part of why I'm good at it. My motivation is internal, but external results contribute to it. The majority of my patients go on with their lives, grateful for the time they were in my care. Knowing this, and having it reiterated when I see them later, is in itself rewarding.

My practice is multi-faceted, and I enjoy the variety. There are some diseases I respond to in my work. I do not have the temperament to do the same thing every day. I'm glad someone does cataract surgery day in and day out, and I congratulate them on their salaries along with their golf course time. But for me, such repetition would be abject misery.

Insurance companies and Medicare are continually trying to cheapen medical services, and through their efforts, they demean the considerable talent and work of dedicated physicians. After investing my life in getting educated to do my job, and then reinvesting it in building my practice and continuing my education, it is painful to be treated as though my work is entry-level. To hear it from them, you might expect a physician to end his patient intake by asking them, 'Would you like fries with that?'

I hold myself to a high standard of self-care. I see it as not only good for me but a part of my social contract with the world I live in and work. I must be able to do my work well and to keep my demands on other's resources to a minimum if I am to know that I am keeping my end of the deal. I also must know that if ever I do require society's resources, in the end, I have given more than I received. Then I would be making myself a successful investment for society, and not a burden."

24.2 The High Standards We Must Follow

"I respect that there are many people who cannot maintain such strict standards. Their mental or physical capacity is just not there, and it is due to reasons they cannot control. This is all the more reason for those of us who are capable of living up to a higher standard to do so.

I do not like getting up at night to take care of someone who is drunk or high and caused an automobile accident, hurting themselves or others. I do not like taking care of people who expect miracles from me after spending a lifetime not taking care of themselves. These people deny any social responsibility in the name of their issues.

Most surgeons get 35 to 40 percent of their income from Medicare. Medicare makes up 60 percent of mine. Private insurance accounts for 25 percent, Medicaid covers 5 percent, and each of those payment sources is quickly losing ground to the fast-growing 5 to 10 percent of patients who have no insurance."

24.3 Decreased Reimbursement and Free Care

"Do you know that doctors are the only professionals in the US that sometimes get paid 180 days after the service? If you try to hire a lawyer, they want money upfront. Then not only are we paid late, but also 60 percent of the reimbursement is canceled or never paid! Incredible!

Doctors all over the country give free care in the name of charity, community service, disease awareness, and to help service organizations reach the highest number of those in need. Our services are also discounted by Medicare and Medicaid. While it is uplifting to be of service to our communities, nothing is redeeming about the losses incurred via Medicare and Medicaid. But the most significant frustration in all of this is that the IRS does not allow us to take any tax deductions for this free or discounted care.

My salary was good. We tend not to reveal our salary because of Stark law II; it is the healthcare corporations that keep us in the dark as well. Like many physicians in this country, my tax bill is not small. Most of us pay more in taxes than a significant portion of working-class America earns. Earning salaries like this means that we can afford to give our children a good education. It means we can invest in our retirements. It means we can be selective about our homes and vehicles. There is a certain amount of privilege that comes with this income, but the income comes with a significant amount of work and dedication. I do not hesitate to say that I earn every penny I make.

Since the introduction of the Affordable Care Act, Congress has been trying to find ways to change healthcare in America drastically. Indeed, healthcare must be available to all who need it. The average American should be able to remain in good health to be a contributing member of society. Legislative in-fighting and half-baked healthcare programs thrown together in last-minute meetings have given many Americans reason to wonder if they will be able to afford to maintain their health. This is irresponsible.

I, too, wonder what will happen when the dust clears. Will doctors be the ones who pay for a new healthcare plan for the country by having our salaries drastically cut? It's hard to believe insurance companies or pharmaceutical companies will have to absorb any losses with their lobbying power. So, while we doctors are doing better than many Americans, it is easy to see where our futures are very much on the line too.

A budding surgeon must be focused. Seeking counsel with the college's pre-med adviser is one of the first things a new student should do. The adviser can steer them to the courses they will need to get into medical school. Without that guidance, it is easy to waste precious scholastic time. It's not that outside interests should not be explored in the classroom as often they help the student maintain their sanity in the high-stress environment that is the pre-med program. It's that specific courses should be taken as early as possible while others are better taken later, and as changes occur, it is the pre-med adviser who will know how best to navigate them.

Maintenance of grades is essential, as is the preservation of reputation. Getting arrested for driving while intoxicated or being involved with a group that endorses violence will severely limit the student's future potential. Most medical schools do background checks on prospective students."

24.4 Difficulties Being a Surgeon and Making Decisions in Seconds

"It is objectively challenging to be a surgeon and make decisions in seconds, while lawyers can sue you and spend thousands of hours evaluating your actions. It is like watching an old football game and criticizing the quarterback for his decision. Why don't you play football? Why don't you come with us to the operating room and see what it looks like saving lives all day long against all the odds?!

After medical school, a general surgery residency is a five-year commitment. It is hard and exhausting work, and by the time a new surgeon is ready to practice as a full-fledged surgeon, they will have been in school and training at least 25 years. While it can be a lucrative living, by the time a surgeon gets their practice up to speed, they're middle-aged. This is not a career for someone motivated solely by the money. A doctor must love what they do. I enjoyed my training, and I would do it again in an instant.

The science and technology that affect surgery are continuously changing, and the changes seem to come faster every year. Patients don't change that much. Their conditions have specific factors unique to each, but their basic needs are much the same. They need to know that I understand where they stand emotionally as well as physically. They need to be able to trust that I am clear about their needs and am capable of responding to them. Finally, they need to feel glad that they came to me after everything is done. I shouldn't have to divide my attention between my patient's needs and the system, which is supposed to enable me to do that.

Legislators are playing the one-upmanship game. Insurance companies are continually changing their billing codes to keep from having to pay for legal services. These irresponsible and unethical practices take some of my attention away from doing the job I am here to do.

Most often, the work I do changes the patient's life. Sometimes my work saves a life. While this is highly rewarding, the other side of the coin is that it is plain wrong for the government and insurance companies to do anything that might even slightly diminish my ability to do my work.

The road to becoming a general surgeon is a hard one, and the number of general surgeons in the United States is dropping each year. Surgeons are becoming more valuable as our numbers decrease. The demand is not falling.

I always start my initial consultation with a patient by talking about the team. Either we work as a team, or we fail. It's that simple.

I maintain a professional standing in my community, a solid rapport with my peers, and I have developed a good reputation with former patients. This is the first thing a new patient will be exposed to before they even know me.

In the initial meeting, I am forthright and assertive, ready to hear them out, and I encourage them to speak their piece. They all seem to comprehend the idea of teamwork, and they all respond well to it. Some take it seriously while others can't look past the idea that I am supposed to fix whatever ails them regardless of what they may do beyond our moments together.

There's nothing I can do about those who don't see the necessity of working together. I can do my best work, give them the information they need to make healthy decisions from that day forward, and offer to be available should they need guidance at any point. If they don't understand the importance of teamwork by this point, my hands are tied."

Suggested Reading

The challenge of running a medical practice. Minute Hack: MH Contributor; 2018. https://minutehack.com/opinions/the-challenges-of-running-a-medical-practice.

John-Henry Pfifferling. The danger of a dysfunctional medical practice. *Family Practice Management.* 2005; 12(5):40-44. https://www.aafp.org/fpm/2005/0500/p40.html.

T. DeAngelis. Are you really ready for private practice? As a new psychologist, starting your own business is no easy feat. Here's advice to smooth the way. 2011. https://www.apa.org/gradpsych/2011/11/private-practice.

E. E. Frezza. *The Business of Surgery.* New York; Cinemed; 2007; ISBN # 978-0-9788890-0-5.

Chapter 25

The Loneliness of a Physician in Moral Distress

In this session we will talk about:

- *How physicians are alone*
- *Loneliness is pain*

25.1 Physicians Are Alone

"I am Janette Silver – vice chair of family practice – I have been listening and absorbing, and I cannot shake the feeling of a deep and severe solitude that accompanies the doctor during his journey. Did you ever feel that?"

"You are correct and right and very sensitive," replied Carlo. "You are not lonely because you are alone. You are lonely because the people around you cannot bring happiness to your heart and your soul. You can be around many people. You can be in the middle of the party dancing, and you still feel alone. This feeling goes back to when I was a teenager. I went to my first party. Most of the time, at the party, I felt that I was by myself. I thought that I was going out for the illusion of having company. But in reality, I was alone. I was lonely many times in my life when I was at school as a teenager because my parents didn't understand what I was doing. They didn't even talk to me much.

Even married, I was often alone. My wife suffered the consequences of marrying an immigrant in that I had trouble adjusting to the routine.

My wife had her family to back her up. With my family in Italy, I had nobody but her, and she could only do so much for me, as her life was filled with our boys.

The demands of a residency are such that I was alone, even while working. It's called a residency for a reason; you reside at the hospital. I was alone in finding work. I was alone in bringing home money. I was alone in deciding how to invest that money, and I was alone in every decision except for those made about my children. My wife was very much there for that.

In my first year of residency, I was in Washington, DC. I left without any friends. I made no enemies either, but I left as alone as I had arrived.

After that, I went to a two-year program as a preliminary in New Jersey. It was pyramidal, and for sure, there were no friends there, and then I wrapped up my last two years in New York. It was there that I established myself, where I graduated alone, as always. My wife was too busy to come to my graduation ceremony after all my sacrifices to get there.

During my two-year fellowship, I was working 18-hour days, 7 days a week. It is impossible to maintain such a schedule for long and remain healthy, but foreign graduates must do it to succeed in the United States. It's closer to slavery than it was to work. The politics in that fellowship were malignant too. I have never missed those years. In that place, loneliness was reinforced.

Finally, as I prepared for my career in Texas, I thought my loneliness might be behind me. The work was rewarding. I was prolific and productive, traveling the world for my work and with my sons. But there was one thing I failed to do. I was unable to truly savor the moment, to take the time to thank God for all I had and to treasure each moment knowing they never can last. Still, I remained alone.

When I learned that I have cardiac disease, I could tell no one. I have an aberrant pulmonary artery. I have light angina and coronary family problems, with circumflex obstruction. However, I am still doing exercise and hiking, no excuses, even though I know that I cannot take care of myself. If I tell any prospective employers, I'll never get hired. My sons were too young to understand or do anything about it, so I didn't burden them. My wife could only worry and make it worse, so I didn't tell her either. I'll need surgery to correct this, and I never have time. I suppose I am a loner by nature. Nobody wants to be lonely, but I don't see a way around it just yet."

25.2 Loneliness Is Pain

"In Brazil, there is a word, 'Saudade,' which does not translate fully into any other language. But it makes me wonder if I may have some Brazilian ancestry. Saudade is a type of melancholy that is not a product of any incidents; instead, it is a natural part of their identity. I have never been complete without my solitude; even when I was busy and productive, I knew it was nearby. The Brazilians embrace this. I don't know if I can.

I often think this disease of loneliness will kill me. I can be so busy I barely have time to sleep. I can be productive and creative, and I can make many things better while receiving deserved accolades, but I know it is nearby, waiting. I understand that some people go into a deep depression and then commit suicide. I've considered suicide, but not from a place of wanting to do it.

There is one good thing that comes from this solitude, introspection. I have gone deep within myself to understand why I feel specific ways, why I do certain things, even simple things, and because of that, I am very comfortable being me. If you look around, you will see that very few people are truly satisfied with being themselves.

There is another view of loneliness. I've read many books about the isolation of the soul. Many authors exploring melancholy have stated that as society has come to move faster and faster, it's easier for the soul to starve. Perhaps this is why there is a mindfulness movement now. Indeed, we must slow down if we are to survive sometimes. Maybe I needed this intense solitude as a sort of convalescent time. Spending my time alone, I have found the freedom I never realized I had been missing."

Suggested Reading

S. Fitch. Does loneliness add to physician burnout? – Yes, and you can fix it. *Med Page Today*; 2019. https://www.medpagetoday.com/publichealthpolicy/generalprofessionalissues/77476.

Alone or together? Addressing physician isolation. 2014. http://hss.semel.ucla.edu/2014/03/alone-or-together-addressing-physician-isolation/.

Isolation and loneliness that physicians experience. 2019. https://www.kevinmd.com/blog/2019/05/the-isolation-and-loneliness-that-physicians-experience.html.

Chapter 26

Divorce as a Consequence of Moral Distress

In this session we will talk about:

- *The divorce rate for physicians being sued*
- *Marriage weak spot*
- *My marriage was not there for me*
- *Vindictive ex-wife*

26.1 Divorce Rate for Physicians Being Sued

"Did you divorce then?" added Dr. Silver. "Why so many divorces?"

Carlo replied, "Dr. Anupam Jena, a hospital physician and an assistant professor at Harvard Medical School, said in a study, 'It's been speculated that doctors are more likely to be divorced than other professionals because of the long hours they keep and the stress associated with the job, but no large-scale study has ever investigated whether that is true. We found that doctors have the lowest rates of divorce among healthcare professionals.' Divorce rates among doctors vary according to specialty.

I was married to a good woman. She was married to a good man. And yet when the stress got too much, we could not stay together. We each did things the other could not deal with. We each felt, at times, like the other did not care even though we both cared deeply the entire time.

While the everyday stresses of a physician's life may not contribute to the divorce rate all that much, a lawsuit can change that dramatically. The divorce rate among physicians who are being sued is estimated to be 90 percent.

Financial realities change drastically during and after a suit, and a family may not be able to maintain the life to which the family has grown accustomed. The change is often sudden, as was the case in our marriage, and it is hard not to feel as if you're under attack from all sides when in the middle of such turmoil.

One thing we were blessed in was that we both love our sons so much that they didn't suffer as many kids do, feeling like they had to take sides.

When I was at my lowest, I was forced by circumstances and decisions that I had been a part of, to maintain two households. My wife returned to Pennsylvania with our boys. I moved to a small East Texas town to eke out a living as best I could. This was the loneliest time I have ever known. My resentment of my wife grew and grew. She had children. She had her family close by, and she had my money. I had a job that was well beneath my skills and didn't fulfill me. I had a constant barrage of legal issues wearing me down every day. I had lawyer's fees on top of all of my other expenses. I wanted her to move back so that we could face this as a family, but she was afraid of all the uncertainties. I tried to find a job near her, but that never happened.

She was a good woman, she was a good wife more often than not, and nobody is good all the time. I did my best to be a good husband to her as well, and I know that I failed her at times. One of the things that has helped us to move forward through this time has been our mutual and indubitable love of our sons. I will always wonder what might have happened had she moved back to stand by me as I fought through those tough times. I like to think that I would have fought harder, and my win would have been more complete. But perhaps it would have brought about a destructive end for us that we could not have worked through. I will never know. After almost three years of separation, I found companionship, and she was upset by that."

26.2 Marriage Weak Spot

"Looking back, it's easy to see that she couldn't handle everything falling around her. She needed to be near her parents at that time. Perhaps I could have saved our marriage by returning to Pittsburgh and taking work outside the medical field, but then I would have been miserable, and that's no way to be in marriage either. I had to move forward, fighting for my career. She had to return to a place where she could feel safe. She is a gentle-hearted woman. This fight could not be hers.

My family had its weak spots, as any family does. Overall, we were active in our love of each other and of our children, we shared dreams for them and us, and we knew what it would take to make those dreams come true. We were devoted to that. But even the most reliable family can be broken.

My wife and I each made some bad choices during that time in our lives. We were not prepared for the stress and the pain, and we could not stand together against it. But I have learned that a brain under extreme duress works differently than a mind that is calm and clear and dispassionate. We were not our usual selves during that time. If we had been, our marriage would still be active. Therefore, I say that we must not judge others when we do not know the context in which they're acting."

26.3 My Marriage Was Not There for Me

"My marriage is not there now. My responsibilities to my family are still very much with me and will remain, but my marriage is decidedly behind me now. Sometimes I wonder if I could go back to it. Could I go back to the life we lived before? Could I go back and create a new life with her?

The marriage had unhealthy aspects. Looking back and seeing it from this distance, I see much that would have to change. Much would also have to be forgiven.

Neither of us ever wanted to hurt the other, but we did in lots of little ways, digging and picking, always feeling like we were right if the other would only see it. Then there was the defensiveness. Each of us feeling attacked, not always responding most maturely. We developed some nasty habits together. I have wondered if we could change those habits.

It was a recurring theme in our marriage. She was not there when I needed her, but the moment I walked away, she became available. I don't walk away until I am done. I graduated from residency. She was not there. I got diagnosed with angina; she was not there. Indeed, she had excuses for every time, but her priorities were clear, and I was not one of them. Maybe it would be better to say that she was the greatest quarterback of the day after! Always one day late to throw the ball. Even when the big lawsuit came, she was not there. She was comfortable close to her parents. And I let her. That was the killing blow for our marriage.

Marriages sometimes end because of tangible elements. Those are money, school, work, housing, and all the physical necessities. Sometimes they end because of the intangible elements. Maybe the love fails a test, perhaps the friendship or the trust dies, perhaps the pride and defensiveness of both parties wear one or both of them down, and they give up staying alive. Money is supposed to be the number one cause of divorce in the country now. If it is, it's because the way each person relates to money shows irreconcilable differences in their values or their emotional capabilities.

Sometimes, when you're down as low as you can get and you don't know how you're going to keep going, life gives you the help you need. People you never thought of will step up and offer a word of encouragement, a helping hand, or a much-needed observation. I think of that as the hand of God reaching out to me through someone. I hope I've been that instrument for someone else.

My distance from her has shown me a bigger world. I am more comfortable with my sexuality, with my relationships with others. Now I get told that I know how to talk to people, this is new! Even with my strong personality, I am getting to be known as a people person. This is in part due to the people I surround myself with, and in part, because I can relax and be myself now. It's also because I've made a practice of learning from everyday people. I've learned a lot about myself and my world by watching them. So, when I ask myself if I could go back, the answer is no. I am a different person than I was then. I will never censor myself to please someone else again. I know she has changed as well. She was a good woman."

26.4 Vindictive Ex-Wife

"She then lost her mind, and she became vindictive and jealous.

She never was able to recognize and take her responsibilities, and therefore she will live in misery. She is so miserable that she tried to have the marriage annulled by the Catholic Church after she divorced legally in court and got 80 percent of our properties and money.

We got married in court in April the same year we divorced, there was no need to get married in the church, but she insisted; do you think the marriage in the church was just a show? We were married by a priest she'd known for 20 years.

Does it mean that either her Church or the Catholic school she attended did not prepare her?

She lived with her mom, dad, brother, and she has uncles, aunts, cousins, all living in the same area. She had very religious aunts and a grandmother in Italy. I was the 'immigrant' alone, not even speaking the language, with nobody to talk to since, in those times, the internet and cell phones were not readily available.

Why did she not ask for the annulment before getting all that money? So, first the money, then God. She blamed her lack of emotional preparation for marrying at the age of 30! Was she really that unprepared? You don't have to get a divorce from court to get an annulment from the Church, and she had planned it all.

She is well-financed, and she does not even go to church to pray or donate. She just used the Catholic Church tribunal as she used me.

She left me alone in Texas for many years, staying in Pittsburgh to enjoy her family and the house, and she never worked during those years. She divorced because she did not want to be close to her husband. She left me while I was fighting a lengthy lawsuit alone.

As a person, she lost her mind, and I hope that the Lord can help her one day to stop with her vindictive and greedy attitude. Maybe she has secondary moral distress as well."

Suggested Reading

E. Izadi. Divorce among doctors isn't as common as you think, study finds. *The Washington Post*, 2015. https://www.washingtonpost.com/news/to-your-health/wp/2015/02/19/divorce-among-doctors-isnt-as-common-as-you-think-study-finds/

D. P. Ly, S. A. Seabury, and A. B. Jena. Divorce among physicians and other healthcare professionals in the United States: Analysis of census survey data. *BMJ*, 2015; 350. doi: https://doi.org/10.1136/bmj.h706; https://www.bmj.com/content/350/bmj.h706.

University Times. *Research Notes.* https://www.utimes.pitt.edu/archives/?p=5326.

Bruce L. Rollman, Lucy A. Mead, Nae-Yuh Wang, and Michael J. Klag. Medical specialty and the incidence of divorce. *The New England Journal of Medicine* 1997; 336:800–803. https://www.nejm.org/doi/full/10.1056/NEJM199703133361112.

J. Marbella. Divorce and the doctor study: That surgeons and psychiatrists have highest rates is no surprise to many in the field of medicine. Others want a second opinion. *The Baltimore Sun*, 1997. http://articles.baltimoresun.com/1997-03-13/features/1997072018_1_divorce-rate.

Wilkinsson and Finkbeiner. Divorce facts and statistics. What affects divorce rates? 2017. http://www.wf-lawyers.com/divorce-statistics-and-facts/.

Chapter 27

The Stress of a Lawsuit Breaks Families

In this session we will talk about:

- *Bringing the moral injury home*
- *Reinventing yourself*

27.1 Bringing the Moral Injury Home

"The pressures of the lawsuit were more than our marriage could handle, however, and between us, we made a few messes. They say that love can fix anything. Perhaps that's true, but only if you let it, and if you can't see how it affects things, it's hard to let go and trust. Neither of us could let go and trust. We partially let go, but we never believed.

The children were a different story altogether. My wife may not have had what it takes to stay with me through better or worse, but she did right by our boys. While I had to remain in Texas to fight this legal battle, I had to work in jobs that were sub-par at best. I had to live in towns with little to no cultural or educational options, and she did right by taking the boys back to Pennsylvania, where my money could get them the education they needed to make something of themselves.

The boys grew up with grandparents, cousins, a diverse culture, and a terrific education thanks to their mom. They turned out to be good kids and are turning into good men as well. I credit her with most of this, and I thank God. But damn, I was lonely!

I don't mean I was just tired of living alone and bored. This wasn't some shallow loneliness used to justify cheating on my wife. My very reason for doing what I did no longer matters in more ways than one. I could not do the work I loved anymore, even though I am excellent at it, and that was one hard pill to swallow. I could not get a colleague to look me in the eye or treat me like an equal. Being a pariah is a curse I would not wish on my worst enemy. I was the subject of gossip for as long as I stayed anywhere. The sidelong looks and the way nurses would talk to me made it clear I was the butt of many a joke. I had to do work that was marginal because of the ancient equipment and politics of small-town hospitals.

Add to this not having my wife and sons to look forward to coming home to. Add to this not playing ball with my boys, not making love with my wife, and only feeling needed for the money I could make.

I was a man whose needs could not be met and who could not churn out money like a machine without support.

My sons and I texted each other frequently. We talked on the phone a lot. I came up with vacations, ski trips, and any other excuses to spend time with them and to create memories of them at specific times in their growth.

They say you should never lean on your children for emotional support. I'm not so sure about that. If you're careful not to burden them too much, it can help them to know you better and to believe in themselves more too. I did not have anybody to talk to except them, and I admit I talked to them too much venting about my marriage problems with them. It was not good! Naturally, they depended on me for advice. We would talk about school, girlfriends, sports, academics, and many of their interests too. Sometimes I gave advice, sometimes I encouraged them, and sometimes I just listened and enjoyed who they were at the moment. My sons, of course, have very different personalities as siblings often do. With my oldest son, I could talk about everything. We pulled no punches, and it has given him a fuller understanding of his father as a human, warts and all, that he can both love and like. My younger son was too young to open up to like this when I first started opening up to them, so we created a different dynamic. We talk more about creativity, philosophy, story writing, and the like. As he has grown, the conversations have opened up more."

27.2 Reinventing Yourself

"From all of this, I found I was reinventing myself. I had become a better father than I had previously known existed. I had created a focus that could make me happy and fill me with joy through my newly created friendships with my sons. I had a sanctuary in my heart from which I could begin my healing journey.

I went to their graduations, but I did not get to see them growing in middle school and high school. I didn't see them getting ready for prom, looking handsome in tuxes with a beautiful girl on their arm. There were no ball games, no sporting events, no hugs, no quiet talks in the evening sitting together. There was no working out together. You really can't teach a child to go to the gym every day from a thousand miles away. I missed all this, and it still hurts.

I didn't have all the beautiful times raising my boys. I adapted and had other beautiful times with them, and we are friends now, so I am blessed and grateful for my loneliness. I'll never know that experience unless I father more children, something I do not expect to be doing.

I paid rent in Texas and a mortgage in Pennsylvania. I moved from one small Texas town to another and another, ad nauseam, trying to stay at least one step ahead of the wolf at the door. Airplane tickets had become a regular expense, and of course, I couldn't be there for emergency decisions.

Some expenses double. Some payments triple, and some costs are wholly new to the situation. A physician must have two cars available in case one breaks down; he has to have a backup. When we were together, her vehicle was my backup. So, there's the expense of one more car. Feeding two households is more expensive than feeding one, even if it's the same number of people. You don't stop to think of all the groceries that are now purchased twice because nothing is shared when there's a thousand-mile gap between kitchens. And of course, when you're living together, it's easy to say, 'be a little careful with this month's grocery budget. Things are a bit tight just now.' You can tell it when they're a thousand miles away, but there's no way to know if she did it or even if she could. Lawyers were necessary at that time. My needs were met on a shoestring. My preference had to be getting my boys raised right at my side.

Even without the pain of divorce, separating a family is hard in several ways, and financially is not the least of them. This killed the family dynamic that fed my soul so richly and put me in total moral distress."

Suggested Reading

Anhedonia. https://www.webmd.com/depression/what-is-anhe
donia#1.

'Lack of Professional Appreciation' tops the list of why physicians
leave. 2013. http://www.phg.com/2013/04/lack-of-professional
-appreciation-tops-the-list-of-why-physicians-leave/.

Tips to survive law suit. https://www.thedoctors.com/articles/youve
-been-served-lawsuit-survival-tips-for-physicians/.

E. Leap. Once upon a time, being a doctor was great. Not anymore.
Kevin MD; 2017. https://www.kevinmd.com/blog/2017/02/upon
-time-doctor-great-not-anymore.html

Chapter 28

The Birth of Moral Distress: The Syndrome

In this session we will talk about:

- *Low satisfaction*
- *The birth of moral injury*
- *The physician is not just a scorecard*
- *Why is moral injury a syndrome?*
- *Physician wellness program*

28.1 Lack of Satisfaction

"This is terrible," the residents and students said in one voice. There was a pause, and then Prof. Heck said, "I am the chair of the ethics committee and an internist by training, I was quiet until now and absorbing the data and your unfortunate experience. I agree with the residents in their comments, but as a grown senior physician, I am growing a sense of unease about the situation. Are you okay? Are we losing good doctors like you? What can we do? Is anything out there tackling these issues?"

"I can share your frustration and worry," Carlo answered. "I do not have a ready answer, but I can tell you what Simon Talbot and Wendy Dean wrote in their article (1).

They reported physicians, like combat soldiers, often face a profound and unrecognized threat to their well-being: moral injury.

Moral injury is frequently mischaracterized. In combat veterans, it is diagnosed as post-traumatic stress; among physicians, it's portrayed as burnout. But without understanding the critical difference between burnout and moral injury, the wounds will never heal, and physicians and patients alike will continue to suffer the consequences."

28.2 The Birth of Moral Injury

"The term 'moral injury' was first used to describe soldiers' responses to their actions in war. It represents 'perpetrating, failing to prevent, bearing witness to, or learning about acts that transgress deeply held moral beliefs and expectations.' Journalist Diane Silver describes it as 'a deep soul wound that pierces a person's identity, sense of morality, and relationship to society.'

The moral injury of healthcare is not the offense of killing another human in the context of war. It is unable to provide high-quality care and healing in the context of healthcare.

Most physicians enter medicine following a calling rather than a career path. They go into the field with a desire to help people. Many approach it with almost religious zeal, enduring lost sleep, lost years of young adulthood, huge opportunity costs, family strain, financial instability, disregard for personal health, and a multitude of other challenges. Each hurdle offers a lesson in endurance in the service of one's goal, which, starting in the third year of medical school, is sharply focused on ensuring the best care for one's patients. Failing to meet patients' needs consistently has a profound impact on physician well-being – this is the crux of consequent moral injury.

In an increasingly business-oriented and profit-driven healthcare environment, physicians must consider a multitude of factors other than their patients' best interests when deciding on treatment. Financial considerations – of hospitals, healthcare systems, insurers, patients, and sometimes of the physician himself or herself – lead to conflicts of interest. Electronic health records, which distract from patient encounters and fragment care, but are extraordinarily effective at tracking productivity and other business metrics, overwhelm busy physicians with tasks unrelated to providing outstanding face-to-face interactions. The constant specter of litigation drives physicians to over-test, over-read, and over-react to results – at times, actively harming patients to avoid lawsuits."

28.3 Physicians Are Not Just Scorecards

"Patient satisfaction scores and healthcare provider rating and review sites can give patients more information about choosing a physician, a hospital, or a healthcare system. But they can also silence physicians from providing necessary but unwelcome advice to patients and can lead to over-treatment to keep some patients satisfied. Business practices may drive providers to refer patients within their systems, even knowing that doing so will delay care or that their equipment or staffing is suboptimal.

Navigating an ethical path among such intensely competing drivers is emotionally and morally exhausting. Continually being caught between the Hippocratic Oath, a decade of training, and the realities of making a profit from people at their sickest and most vulnerable is an untenable and unreasonable demand. Routinely experiencing the suffering, anguish, and loss of being unable to deliver the care that patients need is deeply painful. These routine, incessant betrayals of patient care and trust are examples of 'death by a thousand cuts.' Any one of them, delivered alone, might heal. But repeated daily, they coalesce into the moral injury of healthcare.

Physicians are smart, sturdy, durable, resourceful people. If there were a way to get themselves out of this situation by working harder, more intelligently, or differently, they would have done it already. Many physicians contemplate leaving healthcare altogether, but most do not for a variety of reasons: little cross-training for alternative careers, debt, and a commitment to their calling. And so, they stay – wounded, disengaged, and increasingly hopeless.

I want to make an example of what moral distress can do to you. My youngest son taught me a lesson. We were in a bank, and I got on to one administrator who gave wrong advice to my son. I was right, but my son told me that my reaction was too much, and that guy will remember me at dinner as the asshole who treated him badly during the day. I was not compassionate and definitely too stressed out to realize what I was doing.

Talbot and Dean concluded that to ensure compassionate, engaged, and highly skilled physicians are leading patient care, executives in the healthcare system must recognize and then acknowledge that this is not physician burnout. Physicians are the canaries in the healthcare coalmine, and they are killing themselves at alarming rates (twice that of active duty military members), signaling something is desperately wrong with the system."

28.4 Why Is Moral Injury a Syndrome?

"Moral distress and moral injury are now the same thing as one brings the other, and with the initial injury, the distress starts and never goes away. It is not just a clinical presentation, it is a constellation of symptoms. Therefore, we can define it as a syndrome because it has many causes, many symptoms, and clinical presentations. The following is what I define as moral distress syndrome:

1. PTSD
2. Burnout

3. Empathy
4. Emotional detachment
5. Inability to sustain friendship or family duties
6. Divorce
7. Suicide

The presentation can be a simple discontent with the job, complaint of lack of recognition, or it can start with a lawsuit. The clinical symptomatology can include the following:

1. Headache, fatigue, insomnia, muscle ache and stiffness, heart palpitations, GI syndrome
2. Inability to concentrate, memory loss, confusion, indecisiveness
3. Shock, anxiety, nervousness, depression, anger, frustration, worry, fear, irritability, guilt, shame, insecurity
4. Hyperactivity, change in eating habits, defensive approach with patients, smoking, drinking, yelling, abusive disorders"

28.5 Physician Wellness Program

"According to Talbot and Dean (1):

> The simple solution of establishing physician wellness programs or hiring corporate wellness officers won't solve the problem. Nor will pushing the solution onto providers by switching them to team-based care, creating flexible schedules and float pools for provider emergencies, getting physicians to practice mindfulness, meditation, and relaxation techniques, or participating in cognitive behavioral therapy and resilience training. We do not need a Code Lavender team that dispenses 'information on preventive and ongoing support and hands out things such as aromatherapy inhalers, healthy snacks, and water' in

response to emotional distress crises. Such teams provide the same support that first responders provide in disaster zones, but the 'disaster zones' where they work are the everyday operations in many of the country's major medical centers. None of these measures is geared to change the institutional patterns that inflict moral injuries.

What we need is leadership willing to acknowledge the human cost and moral injury of multiple competing allegiances. We need guidance that dares to confront and minimize those competing demands. Physicians must be treated with respect, autonomy, and the authority to make rational, safe, evidence-based, and financially responsible decisions. Top-down authoritarian mandates on medical practice are degrading and ultimately ineffective.

We need leaders who recognize that caring for their physicians results in thoughtful, compassionate care for patients, which ultimately is good business. Senior doctors whose knowledge and skills transcend the next business cycle should be treated with loyalty and not as a replaceable, depreciating asset."

The auditorium all agree in those last sentences. "Talbot and Dean did a fantastic job in recognizing these issues. Wow," commented Prof. Heck.

Reference

1. Simon G. Talbot and Wendy Dean. Physicians are not 'burning out.' They are suffering moral injury. *Stat News*; 2018. https://www.statnews.com/2018/07/26/physicians-not-burning-out-they-are-suffering-moral-injury/.

Suggested Reading

E. E. Frezza. *Tangled Sutures.* Austin, TX; TMA; 2018. www.texasme
dicalassociation.org.

E. E. Frezza. *Medical Ethics.* New York; Routledge; 2018; ISBN #
978-1-138-58107-4.

E. E. Frezza. *The Miserable Doctor.* Sacramento, CA; Cure Your
Practice Press; 2019; ISBN # 978-1-7047-7-3056.

E. E. Frezza. *The Health Care Collapse.* New York; Routledge; 2018;
ISBN # 978-1-138-58110-4.

Chapter 29

Do Physicians Suffer from Discrimination?

In this session we will talk about:

- *How physicians cannot share the pain*
- *Physician discrimination*

29.1 Physicians Cannot Share the Pain

"Can I ask a question? I am Prof. Gazidis, I am not a doctor, but since the subject was interesting, I came this morning from my college of law to follow the development of this issue in medicine since we were already involved in finding a solution or making suggestions. What is the legal implication of all of this?"

Carlo took a deep breath and said, "Sadly, there is no protection for physicians. One physician who is also a lawyer, Louise B. Andrew, MD, JD, wrote an excellent article on physician suicide on Medscape. She made a few good points which I would like to summarize here (1).

Most states have physician health programs that may or may not be associated with the medical licensing authority, and many have regulations that allow a physician enrolled in a physician health program, who is compliant with treatment, to check 'no' on the mental health questions on licensure applications. However, physicians who are contemplating or in need of treatment are almost universally unaware of such 'safe harbor' provisions (1).

Most physicians assume that any state agency or treating physician will share confidential information about them to the licensing authority. Additionally, any lack of disclosure on an employment or credentialing application can be cited as grounds for termination or removing the credentials."

29.2 Physician Discrimination

"Discrimination in obtaining insurance coverage is prevalent, but the problem with mental illness and physicians is not widely publicized illness. Health, disability, life, and liability insurance may all be denied to a physician who admits to depression.

Even if disability insurance has previously been procured, its use may subject physicians to repeated humiliating and invasive examinations by detached and dubious 'independent medical examiners' for the insurer, whose motivation is to cut company losses. Many physicians affected by mental illness feel that insurers expect them to adhere to the standard pre-scription 'physician, heal thyself.'

Despite the protections afforded by law to citizens and other professionals who have disabilities, the potentially devastating effects triggered by a physician's self-reporting of depression may delay or, in fact, preclude appropriate treatment.

Medical licensure applications and renewal applications frequently require answers to broad-based questions regarding the physician's mental health history without regard to current impairment. The courts have determined that they are impermissible because the resultant examinations and restrictions constitute discrimination under Title II of the Americans with Disabilities Act (ADA) based on stereotypes. However, still, impermissibly broad parameters persist in almost half of all licensure applications' mental health questions."

Reference

1. Louise B. Andrew. What contributes to the high prevalance of physician suicide? *Medscape*; 2018. https://emedicine.medscape.com/article/806779-overview.

Suggested Reading

P. Wible. Why do doctors commit suicide? *The Indian Sun*; 2018. https://www.theindiansun.com.au/2018/10/17/doctors-commit-suicide/.

J. G. W. S Wong. Doctors and stress. *Medical Bulletin*; 2008; 13(6). http://www.fmshk.org/database/articles/03mb1_3.pdf.

E. Lee Vliet. Physician suicide rates have climbed since Obamacare. *Physician News Digest*; 2015. https://physiciansnews.com/2015/05/19/physician-suicide-rates-have-climbed-since.

C. Ceccini. A stigma no physician can afford. *Pediatrics*; 2018. http://bagofpediatricks.com/2018/02/22/a-stigma-no-physician-can-afford.

E. E. Frezza. *Tangled Sutures*. Austin, TX; TMA; 2018. www.texasmedicalassociation.org.

E. E. Frezza. *Medical Ethics*. New York; Routledge; 2018; ISBN # 978-1-138-58107-4.

E. E. Frezza. *The Miserable Doctor*. Sacramento, CA; Cure Your Practice Press; 2019; ISBN # 978-1-7047-7-3056.

E. E. Frezza. *The Health Care Collapse*. New York; Routledge; 2018; ISBN # 978-1-138-58110-4.

Chapter 30

American Medical Association (AMA) Directions

In this session we will talk about:

- *The AMA and moral distress*
- *Physicians are the worst patients*

30.1 The AMA and Moral Distress

"The American Medical Association created a new Physician and Medical Student Suicide Prevention Committee intending to address suicide and mental health disease in physicians and medical students. As per their House of Delegates resolution 959 of the year 2018, their committee will be charged with:

1. Developing novel policies to decrease physician and medical trainee stress and improve professional satisfaction.

2. Repeated and widespread messaging to physicians and medical students, encouraging those with mood disorders to seek help.
3. Working with state medical licensing boards and hospitals to help remove any stigma of mental health disease and to alleviate physician and medical student fears about the consequences of mental illness and their medical license and hospital privileges.
4. Establishing a 24-hour mental health hotline staffed by mental health professionals whereby a troubled physician or medical student can seek anonymous advice. Communication via the 24-hour helpline should remain anonymous. This service can be directly provided by the AMA or could be arranged through a third party, although volunteer physician counselors may be an option for this 24-hour phone service."

30.2 Physicians Are the Worst Patients

"Physicians are also often their own worst doctors and feel they can handle their own health issues and stress. There is the ever-present social stigma about seeking mental health treatment, but for physicians, this is magnified by the fear of being penalized and having their medical license jeopardized if they seek treatment for depression or stress. We encourage others to find mental health professionals if appropriate, but most physicians are afraid to do so themselves because such treatment must be reported on each medical license renewal application, increasing the risk of losing one's license and livelihood. Physicians also fear losing hospital privileges if therapy for depression is disclosed. Hospital administrators increasingly use mandated psychiatric treatment as a bullying tactic to remove independent-thinking, patient-focused physicians from hospital staff. A death by suicide is devastating to families, leaving emotional scars that may never heal. Physicians' family members often have significant support to help with grief and shock, but very little attention is paid to the needs of patients, especially older patients who often have profound feelings of loss, and little support to help them through the unexpected loss of a trusted physician upon whom they depended. Most doctors go into medicine genuinely committed to helping people who are ill and in pain. In the end, they end up with an injury like the young soldier who goes to war for the first time and gets scarred for the rest of his life. This is a moral injury. I hope that God can also help us," concluded Carlo with a deep emotional voice.

The audience was quiet again.

Suggested Reading

E. E. Frezza. *The Health Care Collapse*. New York; Routledge; 2018; ISBN # 978-1-138-58110-4.

AMA 2018 resolution. Proceedings of the 2018 Annual Meeting of the American Medical Association House of Delegates. https://www.ama-assn.org/press-center/press-releases/increasing-awareness-suicide-risks-save-lives.

E. E. Frezza. *Tangled Sutures*. Austin, TX; TMA; 2018. www.texasmedicalassociation.org.

E. E. Frezza. *Medical Ethics*. New York; Routledge; 2018; ISBN # 978-1-138-58107-4.

S. Talbot and W. Dean. Physicians aren't 'burning out.' They're suffering from moral injury. 2018. https://www.statnews.com/2018/07/26/physicians-not-burning-out-they-are-suffering of moral injury.

E. E. Frezza. *The Miserable Doctor*. Sacramento, CA; Cure Your Practice Press; 2019; ISBN # 978-1-7047-7-3056.

American Medican Association. Board of Trustees executive summary. 2019. https://www.ama-assn.org/system/files/2019-04/a19-702.pdf.

Chapter 31

Safe Space and Final Introspections

In this session we will talk about:

- *Needing a circle of friends*
- *Loss of your reputation*
- *Difficult battle*
- *Needing a safe space*

31.1 Needing a Circle of Friends

The dean, the CEO of the hospital, and Jeremy, his friend and the chair of surgery, stood in applause. Jeremy said, "My friend, your life and experience was tough but brought us lots of insight. Did you learn anything from all these bad experiences at a personal level deep in your soul?"

Carlo said, "Passing judgment is far too easy a thing to do. Witnessing a few actions or decisions someone makes, without the possibility of knowing the entire story, attaching motives and values from other times, other places, and other people. Sometimes we don't even know we're doing it.

We may see them as whiners who never make an honest effort to solve their problems, and even seem to want the problem more than the solution. Maybe we see them as losers, leaving themselves at the whim of forces beyond their control and never getting a clue about how to respond to those forces. Perhaps we see them as victims of circumstance, under a cloud that they cannot seem to get clear of, and yet we respect their apparent efforts. All of these judgments are easy to make; however, they all suffer from the same fundamental error. They assume that the human psyche is two-dimensional.

Most of what we do is unconsciously motivated. It's unlikely that anybody sees themselves as wanting to remain a victim.

Slowly life began to fall apart around me. I'm no whiner, and I'm no loser. But I'm not a victim of circumstance either. Now that I have some time between who I am and the crumbling of my life, I can see many contributing factors. But at the moment, all I could see was irresponsible people blaming others for the mess they made, corrupt or lazy attorneys not even ensuring they had a solid case to file, and a good-old-boy system in the medical field that I had no way of accessing, so I got thrown under a lot of buses. When life begins to fall apart around you, it is difficult to remember who you are. Fear sets in quickly, and you can revert to defense mechanisms you learned in childhood, though they are no longer appropriate to your circumstances. It is easy to fear the people you love the most, and trust can fly out the window. All the things you used to take pleasure in don't matter anymore, and you don't know why they ever did. The parts of life that defined your happiness either lose their importance in your life or you wonder why they were taken away from you. Heaven help the person who tells you that you brought any of it on yourself. I had five more years of pursuing happiness before this became the definition of my life."

31.2 Loss of Your Reputation

"Some things will come to matter less and less over time. My reputation with people who are too afraid of the word 'lawsuit' to do the right thing is a good example.

Some things I may be able to recover partially, but family and relationships are difficult. Financially, it was a disaster. Big losses!

Of course, there are new things that will come into my life because of the lawsuit. New cards are being dealt all the time. This leaves the perennial unknown. There will undoubtedly be opportunities I cannot yet imagine. I will always have the drive to learn more, to do more, to discover new things, and that will bring me many opportunities.

Nine years ago, I was dealt a terrible hand. I have been learning how to 'play' it since, and I'm still learning. I'm not leaving the table.

While I cannot control the actions of others, and many of their actions have caused me great pain and cost me much of the things that make my life happy, I can control my responses to them. I can own my past mistakes. Indeed, I could have done things differently, and perhaps there would have been different results. I did what I thought was best. This is the time for me to learn from hindsight."

31.3 Difficult Battle

"A person who can effectively utilize emotional detachment with your own issues can set apparent boundaries. Be it in social situations, during family strife, or in their professional discernment, these people earn great respect for their ability to remain calm and make clear decisions, all the while respecting the emotions of others. For the majority of people, emotional detachment is a far cry from reality. Choosing not to engage when emotions run high seems impossible to most people. Unfortunately, the news media, entertainment sources, politics, and even religious leaders can feed this disempowering lie. If done right, emotional detachment includes empathy. Without empathy, emotional detachment would be cruel. There is a common myth that compassion requires vulnerability. It is only through honest emotional detachment that one can be of service with compassion.

This is the balance a doctor strives for every day. Whether we must give a patient bad news or we are helping them come to an informed decision from an emotionally charged place, we must first empathize, and then we must detach. A doctor must learn emotional detachment, and he must own it completely. Any doctor can find himself in the face of shocking trauma at any time; it's one of the characteristics of the profession. This is a large part of why doctors often have an air of authority and are often seen as wise.

Emotional detachment in empathy allows one space to rationally choose their responses without being drawn into a state of being overwhelmed or manipulated. Emotional boundary management is a useful and common tool. Whether responding to an overwrought patient or an overwhelmed peer, control of emotional boundaries is crucial to maintaining one's integrity, dignity, and choice capacity.

Guilty until proven innocent! That's what it feels like. Guilty until proven innocent is profoundly flawed. Everybody looks at the physician like they are a criminal. It doesn't even matter if the charge isn't all that damning."

31.4 Needing a Safe Space

"I have been looking for a safe space. There have been times that I was bluffing, and I acted like I had a safe space. I remember when this lawsuit began. I went to work back in Texas. All I was looking for was a place to hide. This was a search for a safe space.

If a soldier can rely on the VA system to get treated, and they get disability and other perks, the physician is alone in this battle, left abandoned by the hospital, organization, and medical boards.

We need to set a safety net, private psychological support that cannot be reported to anyone or we will continue to see suicide increase and physicians burning out of practices. I hope this book will help physicians and corporate hospitals to open their eyes to the issues before it is too late.

I was not in a safe place. I never understood what a safe space was. It's not a cave where the bats go to sleep after a night on the hunt. It's not a bank where you put your money. It's not a house with millions of soldiers surrounding you. A safe space is a home with joy, love, and happiness. It took many years to understand that. Only three things can bring you happiness. Family brings happiness; love brings happiness, and relationships bring happiness. Being kind to people brings you joy.

From this safe space, you can forget about the unjust treatment that you received. You can look at the world in a much more constructive and compassionate way. Safe space, there is no safe space. You make a safe space by creating relaxation, happiness, and love.

I have been searching for a long time for that. I am working to create it now, and I feel that I am very close. Maybe I needed to lose my safe spaces so that I could honestly know and appreciate the next one I made. If this is my gift from God, I am grateful."

All the audience stood and applauded Carlo; for several minutes they could not stop clapping and praising. Carlo was emotional. A few tears appeared in his eyes.

Hopefully, his bad experience will serve someone else as well as the new generation of residents and doctors that were still applauding and connecting with him in a long-standing ovation.

The End.

Index